Single-Subject Experimental Designs in Communicative Disorders

Leija V. McReynolds

Professor, Hearing and Speech Department
University of Kansas Medical Center

and

Kevin P. Kearns

Supervisor, Speech Pathology Section
New Orleans Veterans Administration
Medical Center

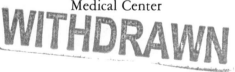

UNIVERSITY PARK PRESS
Baltimore

UNIVERSITY PARK PRESS
International Publishers in Science, Medicine, and Education
300 North Charles Street
Baltimore, Maryland 21201

Composed by University Park Press, Typesetting Division
Manufactured in the United States of America by
R. R. Donnelley & Sons Company

Library of Congress Cataloging in Publication Data
McReynolds, Leija V.
Single-subject experimental designs in communicative disorders.
Bibliography: p.235 Includes index.
1. Communicative disorders—Research—Methodology.
I. Kearns, Kevin P.   II. Title.
RC423.M37   1982   616.85'5027   82-8501
ISBN 0-8391-1714-0   AACR2

Contents

Preface

Investigators in the area of communicative disorders have become increasingly aware of the single-subject approach to treatment research. There are, however, a limited number of texts available to guide researchers who would like to utilize within-subject experimental designs. Moreover, those that are available are from psychology and related fields (Sidman, 1960; Hersen and Barlow, 1976; Kazdin, 1980; Johnston and Pennypacker, 1980) and do not specifically address the complex issues inherent in studying disordered communication. Furthermore, although introductory research design textbooks for speech pathologists and audiologists are available (Silverman, 1977; Ventry and Schiavetti, 1980), their overview format has resulted in a cursory discussion of the single-subject approach to intervention research. Within-subject experimental designs have served as a basis of comparison for the more traditional group experimental design in these texts and discussion of the single-subject approach has been restricted to a few pages. It is not surprising, therefore, that few studies published in journals for professionals interested in communicative disorders have used single-case experimental designs.

Despite a growing interest in within-subject methodologies there has not previously been a detailed presentation of this experimental approach as it relates to communicative disorders. This text was written in an attempt to provide researchers, graduate students, and clinicians with a practical resource for teaching and applying single-subject designs for intervention research in communicative disorders.

A second and perhaps more important rationale also prompted this work. The growing use of single-case experimental research in clinical psychology and special education has demonstrated both the "power" and the elegance of this approach. The applied behavioral research is most appropriate for examining factors that are expected to result in improved performance. Thus, the primary interests of within-subject researchers and professionals concerned with the remediation of communicative impairments are integrally related. Investigators using single-case experimental designs attempt to determine what factors can be used to alter a chosen target behavior. Once indentified, these variables can be incorporated into therapeutic programs which are utilized to modify these same behaviors in the clinical setting. In this sense, single-subject research is applied research that has direct clinical application.

A potential benefit of increased use of this experimental approach is related to the issue of accountability. There has been an increasing demand by the consumers of clinical services and by third party funding agencies that professionals demonstrate the effectiveness of their treatment programs. Because within-subject research is treatment oriented, its application by investigators interested in communicative disorders may result in information that will assist clinicians in becoming more accountable. Clinicians may, for example, be able to use the results of carefully controlled studies of individuals to assist them in formulating an efficacious treatment program for clients with similar characteristics.

The behaviors of communicatively impaired individuals and the manner in which they effect and interact with experimental procedures provided additional impetus for the writing of this text. To date, the application of single-subject research designs in communicative disorders is the exception rather than the rule. Researchers have begun to recognize the potential advantages of this approach over traditional methodologies. Yet, because of the infrequent use of the designs in this area, the range of problems that interested investigators face is not yet fully understood. Much of what is known about an applied behavioral approach to communicative disorders research is the result of the logical generalization of principles and procedures that have been effective in other fields such as clinical psychology. It seems likely, however, that the unique challenges encountered in adapting within-subject research designs to the investigation of the behaviors of communicatively impaired individuals will require novel or modified solutions based on the actual use of these designs and the collection of empirical data. Throughout this book examples have been chosen from the communicative disorders literature in an attempt to highlight the methodological issues particular to this field of study. In addition, the presentation of the basic design principles within the context of selected examples might promote an understanding of the single-subject research approach for speech pathologists, audiologists, special educators, psychologists, and other individuals interested in communicative disorders. If successful, this approach might also provide impetus for additional and novel uses of single-subject methodologies in these disciplines. We hope that the subsequent accumulation of data will contribute to the development of an applied behavioral science of communicative disorders.

One of the purposes of *Single-Subject Experimental Designs in Communicative Disorders* is to describe components basic to all single-subject experimental designs. To this end, the first chapter differentiates single-subject descriptive studies from single-subject experimental studies, and the two basic and most frequently used within-subject designs, reversal and multiple baseline, are explained in Chapters 2 and 3. Suggestions for evaluating relevance of data obtained in within-subject studies are presented in Chapter 4; and Chapter 5 covers reliability and the importance of reliability measures.

Another purpose of the book is to expose the reader to new developments and issues in single-subject research. Therefore, discussions of relatively unexplored experimental designs, and issues not previously integrated into a text accessible to students and researchers are presented in Chapters 6 and 7.

We are grateful to the students who have been enrolled in the single-subject research seminar offered in the Hearing and Speech Department at the University of Kansas Medical Center. Over the years they have proposed and encouraged writing a text such as this. Many of the issues raised in the book had their inception in discussions generated by study proposals in the seminar. The students are too numerous to name, but we hope they recognize their input in reading the context of this text.

Other individuals have contributed to this work. We wish to thank June Miller, Chairman of the Hearing and Speech Department, and the other faculty members for their cheerful support during the two-year preparation of the manuscript. A special thank you to Dixie Albert for her patience in typing many revisions of this manuscript and to all the student assistants for compiling files of references and running down needed information. Special gratitude is also offered to Geri Kearns by both of us, for cheerful acceptance of the time needed to complete the task and for her support of the project.

Single-Subject
Experimental Designs
in Communicative Disorders

Preliminaries to Single-Subject Experiments

1

This text discusses experimental research in which variables are manipulated, not just observed, and their effects on other variables are measured (Campbell and Stanley, 1966). Experimental research contrasts with descriptive and correlational research which essentially *describe* or correlate what is observed, but in which no manipulation of variables occurs. There are two broadly defined approaches to experimental research; one is through group designs and the other is through within-subject designs, more familiarly known as single-subject designs. This book is devoted to within-subject experimental research.

Researchers employing within-subject designs are not, however, a breed apart in their view of science and concepts of what constitutes the scientific method from researchers relying on other kinds of designs. All researchers applying the scientific method are empiricists who believe that human behavior is lawful and orderly. They search for this lawfulness through carefully controlled manipulation to discover variables demonstrating a cause-and-effect relationship with the behavior studied. Application of the scientific method, therefore, dictates that all experimental designs, whether they are group or single subject, be founded on the same principles. The difference between group and within-subject designs lies in the manner in which the principles are put into operation in designing studies.

It is not the purpose of this book to introduce the student to attitudes of science or the scientific method. That information is available in numerous texts (Silverman, 1977; Campbell and Stanley, 1966; Siegel, 1956; Guilford, 1954; Winer, 1962; Lindquist, 1953; and Ventry and Schiavetti, 1980), so prior exposure to the basic concepts is assumed. Yet the elements composing the scientific method are fundamental to all experimental research, and before specific components of any one approach can be comprehended an understanding of the basic components should be established. Therefore, a brief review of a few important components of the scientific method precedes the topic of single-subject designs. The review concludes with a comparison of the components as they are used in single-subject and group designs. It is hoped that such a comparison will clarify the rationale, strategy, and designs used in single-subject research.

SCIENTIFIC METHOD COMPONENTS

The scientific method defines criteria for facets of an experimental study. Because many of these are discussed in detail in forthcoming chapters, only a few principles are presented briefly here. The components discussed include: operational definitions, dependent variable, independent variable, control, and reliability.

Operational Definitions

Often investigators wish to explore abstract and theoretical concepts, for example, auditory processing. The scientific method requires that observable, overt units be used in defining the stimuli, behavior, and events involved in an experimental study because data must be obtained to support any conclusions reached. It is not possible to study "auditory processing" unless it is described by operations that can be defined objectively. Defining the concept with an overt, measurable unit gives the concept an operational definition. The units are not the concept itself, but represent the concept or part of it. For instance, an investigator interested in auditory processing may study subjects' perceptual performance when presented with various lengths of sound sequences (CV, CCV, CCVC, etc.). In this case auditory processing represents the behavior studied. It is defined by specifying the contexts of a number of stimulus items and how the subject responds to the stimuli. Suppose that the subject's response is defined as a button press and a correct response is defined as pressing the button enough times to match the number of consonants and vowels in each stimulus item. Each button press results in a mark on a graph paper. These marks would constitute data concerning the subject's perceptual performance. These marks, then, represent auditory processing as defined operationally by the investigator.

No concept is described uniquely by a single operational definition. Instead, many definitions are possible; and the choice depends on which aspects the investigator wishes to study. Thus, auditory processing might be operationally defined by another investigator as a same or different response to pairs of phonemes presented through earphones. Sometimes operational definitions are derived from definitions used by other investigators studying the same behavior or concept, but often each investigator arbitrarily selects measures that suit the events he or she wishes to explore.

Operational definitions are crucial to scientific investigations, not only for gathering objective data, but also to allow replication of the experiment by other investigators. If subjective, abstract definitions are used, other investigators would interpret them from their own viewpoint, which could be different from the original definition. If this were to occur, replications would be impossible.

The development of operational definitions ensures that appropriate measures will be used. Responses defined to be readily discriminable from other subject behaviors increase accuracy of measurement. Operational definitions, therefore, are used to specify both the behaviors that can be measured accurately and the procedures used to measure them. Operationally defined variables and procedures facilitate reliability of the data obtained, and therefore, facilitate conclusions regarding results of the study.

Reliability

Operational definitions are also important to the concept of reliability. Reliability concerns a wide range of factors, which are discussed in some depth in chapter 5. In behavioral or treatment research involving human judgments about subject responses, it is necessary that the judgments be objective. Objectivity is checked by an observer who makes independent judgments of the subject's responses. The degree to which two or more observers agree on the subject's responses is an index of how objective the judgments are, and the confidence with which the reported data can be accepted. There are many forms of reliability and a number of ways to compute it, yet it is an essential component of all research, experimental as well as descriptive. Without reliability data an experimental study reverts to an unconfirmed observational description.

Dependent and Independent Variables

The dependent and independent variables are treated together because of their relationship. The dependent variable is the behavior (or the response) that is measured during the experiment to determine if behavior changes. The independent variable is manipulated by the experimenter to explore if it will effect changes in the behavior (the dependent variable). An example of the two variables may be illustrated by a study of the effect of noise on speech discrimination. The dependent variable is the subject's performance on speech discrimination tasks and the independent variable is the introduction of noise during the task. The importance of operational definitions of the dependent and independent variables cannot be overemphasized. That is, the exact nature of the discrimination task must be specified clearly, as must the nature of the noise introduced during performance on the tasks. Needless to say, the purpose for designing an experimental study is to try to isolate the effect of the independent variable from all the other variables that may influence the subject's performance before and during the experiment. The experimenter designs the study so that extraneous variables are either accounted for or controlled and will not interfere with the effect of the independent variable on performance.

Control

It is primarily in an effort to prevent extraneous variables from confounding the effect of the independent variable that the concept of control enters in to the design of an experimental study. In a sense, all components of an experimental study are designed to isolate the effect of the independent variable. The experimenter recognizes, particularly in a treatment study, that the subject is exposed to a variety of stimuli outside the experimental room during the course of the study, and that time is passing from the moment the subject entered the experiment to termination of the experiment. It is also realized that each subject comes with his or her own history and the history may influence how the subject performs in the experiment. These, and many other variables may interfere with the independent variable effect, preventing a clear-cut investigation of treatment.

The design of the experiment is structured to control for a number of these confounding variables. It is in this regard that group and single-subject designs differ: not in the need for controls, but in the way in which controls are designed into the experiment. Group studies may take several forms, but the basic design includes a large population of potential subjects from which two groups are formed: an experimental group, and a control group. The independent variable is administered to the experimental group but not the control group. Usually subjects in both groups are measured on the dependent variable before the experiment is started and again when the experimental treatment for the experimental group is terminated. Data from all the subjects in both groups are pooled and a mean score is computed. The mean score from the experimental group is compared with the mean score of the control group. If a difference is found, the difference is submitted to a statistical test to determine if the difference in scores between the two groups is significant, or "real." If it is, the experimenter may conclude that the independent variable had an effect on the subjects' performance. Extraneous variables in group designs are controlled by forming a group of subjects, drawn from the same population as the experimental subjects, into a control group receiving only the pre- and post-treatment measures and not the treatment itself. The control group's performance demonstrates that time, maturation, and all the stimuli present outside the experimental environment do not have an effect on subjects' response to treatment. It is assumed that those same variables are acting upon both groups during the experiment, and if the control group's behavior does not change during this time and the experimental group's behavior does, then the change must be due to introduction of the independent variable. Similarly, because the subjects for both groups were drawn randomly from a large population with different histories, both groups probably contained a variety of histories, thus history as a confounding variable could be ruled out. Finally, the statistical test helps the experimenter to look beyond the variability found in examining the individual performances of subjects within each group. Thus, idiosyncratic behavioral patterns are ignored by pooling subject data and the statistic serves as a control for extraneous variables. Naturally, there is a great deal more to the concepts underlying the rationale and components of experimental group designs (Siegel, 1956; Guilford, 1954; Winer, 1962; Lindquist, 1953). This has been a somewhat simple explanation of the controls used in group designs. The intention of this book is not to describe group designs in depth, but to give a general notion of the controls used in group designs compared to those used in within-subject designs. There is a difference in the basic rationale concerning appropriate controls, the kind of data collected, and how data are treated. There is no right or wrong attached to the differences; researchers simply employ the methodology with which they are most comfortable.

In single-subject designs there is no control group; that is, each subject goes through both a no-treatment and a treatment period. The dependent variable (the behavior to be treated) is observed and measured for a period of time before introduction of the independent variable (the treatment). When the behavior has been measured sufficiently to demonstrate that it has not changed during the no-treatment period, the treatment is introduced while measurement of performance continues. After a period of time the treatment is stopped, but the behavior continues to be observed and measured. Thus, each subject goes through all conditions of the study, the no-treatment conditions and the treatment conditions. This is in contrast to group designs in which the control group is never administered treatment and the experimental group receives the treatment but does not go through a period of no treatment. Each group receives only one of the conditions, either no treatment or treatment, but not both. Control in single-subject studies is within the subject; hence the name *within-subject* experimental designs. It is assumed that maturation, time, and other stimuli present in the environment could affect performance during treatment. If this does happen, it would not be possible to attribute behavioral changes to the treatment alone. The rationale is that these variables are present in all conditions, not just during treatment. They are also present during the period in which no treatment is administered. Therefore, if they influence performance in treatment they would also influence performance when treatment is absent. But if behavior changes only when treatment is introduced, not when it is absent, then it is highly likely that the extraneous variables were not affecting the behavior. More specific and detailed explanations of controls inherent in within-subject designs are presented in the next two chapters.

In summary, all scientists adhere to certain principles inherent in the scientific method. There are similarities and differences among researchers using group and single-subject designs. Control components form the greatest differences and these are reflections of philosophical as well as methodological differences. The important agreement is in the insistence that investigators adhere to the components which make experiments profitable to the advancement of scientific knowledge. In the case of treatment research the knowledge additionally advances effectiveness of intervention in treating disordered populations.

Now that the basic components of the scientific method have been reviewed briefly and use of the components in group and single-subject designs has been compared, attention can turn exclusively to within-subject experimental designs.

ADVANTAGES OF WITHIN-SUBJECT DESIGNS

Traditionally, researchers in communication disorders have relied on group and statistical designs to explore treatment variables. In a more recent development, psychology has offered an alternative methodology with certain advantages for investigation of behavioral treatment variables. The methodology is experimental and has been referred to by a number of terms; most common among them are *functional analysis research, the experimental analysis of behavior, single-subject research designs, single-case experimental designs,* or *within-subject experimental designs.*

Interest in this methodology has been growing in diciplines whose major commitment is development of effective and efficient training programs. Adoption of the methodology has been more widespread in psychology by researchers dealing with a wide range of aberrant or deficient behaviors interfering with learning appropriate or socially acceptable skills, or for teaching basic skills to mentally retarded individuals, than in professions dealing with problems involving complex and subtle communicative behaviors. The difference, however, may lie less in the kinds of behaviors dealt with, than in the scientific backgrounds of the professionals in these disciplines.

Be that as it may, intervention researchers are recognizing that single-subject research designs may open up opportunities for conducting treatment studies that have hitherto been beyond their capabilities for a number of reasons. Undoubtedly, there are advantages in using within-subject research designs that can be appreciated by individuals working with disordered populations.

Of considerable value is the fact that experimental studies with single subjects are designed with the needs of the interventionist in mind. That is, the designs are suited to exploring the effectiveness of events used in treating disordered populations. A more accurate statement about suitability is that the designs were developed specifically for that purpose. The label *experimental analysis of behavior* indicates that the focus is on exploring variables responsible for changing behavior, the accepted focus of remediation. Further, the exploration is not correlational, but experimental, which means that the designs will allow cause and effect statements about the dependent and independent variables, statements regarding the functional relationship between treatment variables and behavior changes.

Two other advantages of using within-subject research designs include an opportunity to explore treatment variables on the population requiring the treatment, and freedom to conduct studies with small numbers of subjects. The two advantages interact, of course, because at times group studies requiring large numbers of subjects may prohibit conducting treatment studies, simply because the population is not available. It is difficult to find groups of homogeneous subjects with a similar disorder in one setting, or even several settings, a requirement for well controlled group studies. Seldom does a researcher have available a sufficiently large population to select enough subjects meeting criteria for the studies. Undoubtedly, problems in obtaining an adequate sample of subjects have forced some researchers to abandon treatment research altogether, or have compelled them to shift to exploring treatment variables in normal subjects by disguising the dependent and independent variable in some way (e.g., use of nonsense words or foreign words in speech studies). Generalizing results from normal subjects to disordered populations is not always profitable.

These problems have been partly solved with the introduction of within-subject research designs. Because the subject serves as his own control, finding homogeneous groups of subjects is less crucial. For instance, to prevent subject characteristics from acting as a possible confounding variable, group designs require an experimental group plus a group of similar subjects who never receive the treatment to serve as a control. In single-subject designs, however, each subject is administered all conditions of the experiment. If subject characteristics threaten to form a confounding variable, they would function in this manner in all conditions in single-subject designs, thus cancelling the possibility of confounding the treatment effect. In essence, control is shifted from a control group to a single subject who goes through the no-treatment and treatment phases as often as the design requires. Within-subject control reduces the number of subjects required to conduct a treatment study, and in turn allows researchers to study disordered populations with greater frequency. This is not to say that group studies of disordered populations are impossible and should be abandoned; on the contrary, they continue to be conducted. The number of treatment studies can be increased, however, if single-subject designs are used.

Other properties of within-subject designs make them attractive for treatment research, particularly for carrying out communicative disorders treatment research. One is the nature of the designs. They permit recording behavioral changes in a detailed manner during treatment; a luxury not frequently found in group studies which are commonly one or, at the most, a few treatment sessions in length and involve only one experimental condition. Conversely, often in within-subject designs each response is counted as a data point so that changing patterns in response frequency, whether gradual, rapid, or variable, present a complete profile of the effect of the independent variable on behavior in all experimental conditions. Single-subject designs are time-series designs; behavior is measured over time in all conditions of the experiment. Analyzing temporal behavioral patterns provides the experimenter with meaningful information about procedural efficiency in treatment, information useful for modifying procedures and increasing treatment effectiveness.

As noted, careful documentation of ongoing treatment is not customary in group studies. Neither are displays of raw data; that is, individual data points are habitually not presented for visual inspection in the results. Mostly, performance data from all individuals in a group are pooled and a mean computed to represent an "average" client's performance. Individual variability is recognized; but results, if they reach significance levels, apply to a hypothetical average subject. Considerable attention has been directed to the clinical usefulness of averaged data (Hersen and Barlow, 1976), and an in-depth discussion in these pages will not be attempted. The major point is that there are no "average" clients; therefore, a treatment applicable to an average disordered client is seldom effective for treating clients with characteristics and behaviors different from average.

Within-subject designs do not eliminate the individual variability observed in group studies, but neither do they obscure it. Instead, the studies are designed to reveal individual differences when they exist, so that an experimenter can isolate variables reponsible for the differences, and submit them to experimental evaluation in the hope that they may eventually be eliminated or brought under experimental control. The attitude of researchers using single-subject designs is that individual variability not only exists, but is prominent; therefore, effective treatment programs can be developed only when the variables responsible for client variations are understood and brought under control.

Thus, the growing body of literature on treatment effectiveness attests to advantages in using within-subject designs. These advantages include the ability to use a small number of subjects selected directly from the disordered population to which the treatment applies, and an in-depth analysis of behavioral changes during treatment. Depending on the research background of individual researchers, disadvantages can also be listed as, for example, reluctance to generalize results from a single subject to groups. A number of issues central to deciding the scientific relevance of data have been raised concerning the value of group versus single-subject research to the understanding and treatment of disordered populations. These issues are peripheral to the purpose of this book, but discussions can be found in other sources (e.g., Hersen and Barlow, 1976; Kazdin, 1976, 1978, 1981; Kratochwill, 1978). The emphasis of this text is on explanation of within-subject designs for those desiring to use them. Otherwise, the choice between single-subject and group designs is an individual matter. Both kinds can provide empirical evidence of scientific importance.

DESIGNS IN SINGLE-SUBJECT STUDIES

Although the book is devoted to single-subject experimental research, it seems appropriate to describe other uses of single-subject designs as reported in the literature and to demonstrate that all single-subject studies are not *experimental* studies. Not all single-subject studies are capable of examining cause and effect relationships. Other functions can best be demonstrated by referring to examples of other kinds of single-subject studies in the literature to describe their designs and procedures. These studies differ from the *experimental* study and from each other in the manner and extent of their use of components of the scientific method.

Scientific Method Components and the Single-Subject Design

Single-subject experimental designs customarily are depicted by using the letters *A* and *B*. The A condition refers to the phase in which the behavior to be treated (the dependent variable) is measured a sufficient number of times to assure that it is not changing for other reasons before administration of treatment (the independent variable). The A phase in within-subject experimental designs is referred to as the *baseline*. The B condition follows the A condition and depicts the period during which the treatment is introduced and its effect on the behavior measured. In single-subject experimental designs the B may be followed by another A phase in which the treatment from B is removed to determine if the behavior reverts to the same level as it had been in the first A. (The design then becomes an A-B-A design.) If it does, the effect of the independent variable has been demonstrated in a controlled manner. That is, the behavior changed when treatment was introduced and changed again when treatment was discontinued. Thus, the independent variable was responsible for changes, not all the other variables present during the A and B phases.

A number of modifications are possible in within-subject designs, and these will be discussed at length in ensuing chapters. That is, not all studies employ an A-B-A design. For now, it is only necessary that the basic form is understood for the purpose of comparing other single-subject designs. Keeping in mind that the experimental designs consist of at least one sequence of A-B-A phases to demonstrate experimental control, it is possible to examine other single-subject designs with this standard in mind using the letters A and B. Using the A and B designations and definitions of each given above, it is possible to give a representation of the conditions involved in different forms of single-subject studies and the purpose of each. Furthermore, the A-B designation and knowledge of what is included in each condition is useful for determining how many of the components in the scientific method are present in each kind of single-subject study. Hopefully, the presentation will make comparison of single-subject experimental designs with the other single-subject designs easier. The various designs for single-subject studies are presented in Table 1.

The A-Only Study   Strictly speaking, these studies, although they involve only one subject, are not planned as treatment studies. They are descriptive studies in which a behavior (or behaviors) is carefully described as it occurs in the natural environment. Prominent in this group are the diary

Table 1. Examples of some single subject study designs

Letter(s)	Kind of study	Conditions of study
A	Descriptive	Baseline only, no treatment
B	Descriptive	No baseline, treatment only
AB	Descriptive	Baseline, treatment
ABA	Experimental	Baseline, treatment, baseline
ABAB	Experimental	Baseline, treatment, baseline, treatment

studies of children in the process of language acquisition. This is not the only environment in which descriptive studies are conducted, but customarily the investigator wishes to interfere as little as possible with ongoing events. It is labeled an A study in this text because it bears some resemblance to the A phase in single-subject research in that the occurrence of a behavior is measured in a single subject. It differs from the A phase in a single-subject experimental design in that the behavior is not measured in a carefully structured environment in a controlled manner, and usually several parameters of the behavior are involved in the description (e.g., in language, describing use of pronouns, copula verbs, plurals, etc.). In many instances in a single-subject longitudinal descriptive study it is desirable not to structure the environment and to refrain from introducing any controls. The purpose is to observe and record the behaviors as they occur naturally. For this reason, extraneous variables are not controlled and the investigator makes himself as unobtrusive as possible, simply recording the occurrence of the behavior of interest in a concise manner for later analysis.

An example of a single-subject descriptive study (A study) is one conducted by Baltaxe and Simmons (1977). The investigators obtained samples of an autistic child's spontaneous speech by recording bedtime soliloquies. The study had several purposes: 1) to analyze the language grammatically, 2) to compare differences in the grammatical forms of the autistic child with forms of normal children as reported in the literature, and 3) to explore how much of the child's speech was propositional and how much echolalic. The authors were particularly interested in attempting to discover what role echolalia plays in deviations from normal processes in language acquisition of autistic children, and how far this information can be used in developing therapy programs. The possibility that they wished to explore, as stated in the report (Baltaxe and Simmons, 1977), was: "The child is unable to develop rule-governed speech in the normal fashion. More functional speech behavior develops based on echolalia by processes which may be different from those observed in normal development" (p. 377).

One 8-year-old autistic girl was studied. The child's physical and social history was summarized by the authors in the subject description section of the report. The child's behaviors were itemized but quantitative data from measures used to identify the behaviors were not included in the report. The subject description ends with several descriptive statements such as, "At the time of the present study, when the patient was eight years old, her verbal interactions, insofar as they existed at all, were primarily of an echoic nature" (p. 379), and "She generally demonstrated impairment in interpersonal relationships, which was manifested by aloofness, decreased physical contact, and poor eye contact" (p. 380). It was mentioned that formal psychological and language testing was not attempted because the child was not cooperative.

The procedure for obtaining the samples included placing a tape recorder outside the bedroom door and a microphone in the child's room. The samples were made after the child had gone to bed, the bedroom door had been closed, and the lights turned off. Data for the results consisted of three 45-minute tapes that were phonemically transcribed by a linguist experienced and trained in the work. The linguist apparently checked the accuracy of the transcriptions by comparing the audiotape with the transcriptions a number of times. Data derived from the transcriptions included analysis of the samples regarding propositional versus echolalic speech, grammaticality, and discourse analysis.

Separation of the utterances into propositional and echolalic speech was given to six raters working independently. These same raters also separated the grammatical from the ungrammatical utterances, and then analyzed the type of ungrammatical forms that occurred. The discourse analysis was performed, but Baltaxe and Simmons do not note who completed the analysis or how it was done.

In the results the authors indicate that the six raters disagreed with each other about separation of propositional and echolalic speech to such an extent that it was not possible to report on this purpose. Therefore, the analysis emphasized study of the ungrammatical utterances and results are reported from this analysis primarily. For this report, only the utterances that had been unanimously rated as ungrammatical were analyzed. Data for the results were reported according to categories into which the utterances appeared to fall, five categories in all. The categories were labeled, for example, "utterances in which syntactic co-occurrence constraints were broken," or "utterances in which semantic co-occurrence constraints were broken," and so on. Rather than presenting quantitative data for these categories, the authors presented a few examples of the utterances falling within each category; that is, their interest was in presenting qualitative, not quantitative data.

The purpose of comparing the autistic child's grammar and discourse with normal children's acquisition of grammar was accomplished by examining data from soliloquies of a normally developing child as reported in the literature. Examination of the data led the authors to the following conclusions. 1) It is likely that the data consisted primarily of delayed echolalia rather than propositional speech. 2) The autistic child, like the normal child, appeared to engage in pattern practice and seemed to take pleasure in the sounds of language and manipulation of linguistic units. 3) No evidence of alternations in dialogue between speaker and listener occurs as it does in normal children. 4) The autistic child structures her discourse using processes similar to the processes used by normally developing children. 5) However, the autistic child used the processes in a manner different from the normal subject. The summary conclusions were that the echolalic autistic child develops language by means of linguistic strategies that may be different from normal strategies, and that the analysis supported the authors' "initial hypothesis that the echolalic autistic child appears to develop a limited but usable linguistic system which is based on echolalia" (p. 392). They indicate that the results support language therapy programs based on and incorporating existing echolalic patterns.

Presence of Scientific Components   Naturally, emphasis is placed on different components of the scientific method in descriptive and experimental studies. The purpose for the two kinds of studies is different. In a descriptive study the investigator wishes to describe an ongoing behavior in detail, sometimes in order to identify possible variables for experimental manipulation. Descriptive studies do not allow cause and effect statements; they are not designed to allow them. Therefore, the components important in descriptive studies are those that will enhance obtaining valid and reliable descriptive data. Of the components discussed earlier, operational definitions, reliability, and, to a certain extent, control assume importance in descriptive studies. Other lesser components not included in the discussion of scientific methodology may also be emphasized. The discussion herein is restricted to the components listed in the previous section of the chapter.

The need for operational definitions is exemplified in the problem encountered in the Baltaxe and Simmons study in attempting to separate the child's utterances into delayed echolalic and propositional categories. Because of a lack of operational definitions that could be used by all raters, the attempt had to be abandoned. Consequently, the authors chose to assume that most of the utterances consisted of delayed echolalia, partly on the basis of the child's lack of spontaneous verbalizations during the day. Aside from the problem of categorizing the utterances, the authors chose to use definitions that had previously been used by investigators studying normal language acquisition, a proper choice.

It is less easy to judge the reliability of the data because no independent transcriptions of the utterances were made; however, after the tapes were transcribed, only utterances that were unambiguously rated as ungrammatical by all raters were included in the language analysis. Discarding items not agreed upon is one way to achieve reliability.

Because descriptive studies are frequently attempts to study behavior in as natural a setting as possible, the controls used in descriptive studies may be somewhat different from controls used in experimental studies. In descriptive studies, the controls concern the manner in which data are recorded and analyzed rather than the experimenter or the structure of the environment. However, procedures are usually kept constant for sampling and the data are treated in a detailed way. Constancy of the language sampling was demonstrated in the Baltaxe and Simmons study, although no data on the size of the sample used in data analysis were presented. Therefore, it is difficult to know how large a sample was used for drawing conclusions.

Descriptive studies of a single subject limit the degree to which one may generalize to all subjects with the same disorder. Differences in autistic children are well documented, and the sample obtained from this one child may have been specific to that child, the particular environment in which she lived, and other events in her life. In other words, although a descriptive study of a single subject can provide useful information concerning the presence of a behavior, it will not allow statements regarding general development or generalization to other subjects with similar problems. A descriptive study can offer only speculations regarding the relevance of the data to treatment. This is because the variables suggested as important (as, for example, the Baltaxe and Simmons study suggested that language therapy programs should be based on and incorporate existing echolalic patterns) have not been tested in the study to determine if they have any influence on the behavior when they are applied. Rather than applying the treatment with the assumption that it is the relevant variable, it is necessary first to put it to experimental test. Only results from the experiment can indicate whether it is a useful treatment variable.

The example of a single-subject descriptive study was presented at some length to demonstrate that it is not the same as a single-subject *experimental* study. Not only are the components used in the designs different, but the purpose of the descriptive study is different from the purpose of the single-subject experimental study. Conclusions reached in a single-subject descriptive study are limited to the subject studied primarily because there are no controls for confounding variables that are present and could be influencing the data obtained.

The B-Only Study   Probably the most common single-subject study reported in the communicative disorders literature is the B study describing a treatment. These studies may take several forms from detailed descriptions of a treatment to a general overview of the intent in treatment. Customarily, the behavior to be treated is not measured before treatment; or alternatively, other behaviors indirectly related to the specific behavior treated are measured with standard tests. Often authors also report on the behavior to be treated from subjective observations. Rarely are objective, quantitative data obtained on the occurrence of the behavior before treatment. This lack of a baseline (an *A*) makes comparisons impossible, and without a comparison changes cannot be ascribed to any one variable. The effectiveness of the treatment cannot be substantiated because no data on the status of the behavior before treatment are available. Moreover, in B studies treatment may consist of several steps or phases and subjects are administered all of them in se-

quence. This creates problems if one wishes to determine how much individual phases contribute to the entire treatment, or if each phase must be
administered to obtain behavioral changes. Inasmuch as objective post-
treatment measures may also be absent, results of B studies are frequently
uninterpretable.

The purpose of B studies is not readily apparent; possibly they describe
intervention procedures or programs for others to apply in treating clients
with similar disorders. Sometimes this goal is risky because authors may im-
pute behavioral changes to the intervention procedures without submitting
scientific evidence in support. To conclude that a treatment is responsible for
changing a specific behavior it is necessary 1) to measure the specific behavior
objectively and at length to establish that it is not occurring before treatment,
2) to control for the influence of extraneous variables on the behavior during
treatment, and 3) to use the same objective measure of the behavior during
the entire course of the study. These are the minimum requirements, and
there are others, if an investigator wishes to demonstrate the effectiveness of
an intervention procedure. Furthermore, statements regarding the contribution of each step in a program require that steps be evaluated independently
and in combination with the other steps—a time-consuming project.

The B-only study is exemplified in a report by Brookner and Murphy
(1975) on teaching a nonverbal child to communicate. A number of factors
could be examined in this study, but the discussion will be restricted to factors aiding in distinguishing B designs from single-subject experimental
designs.

The first concern in the Brookner and Murphy study was measurement
of the behavior to be trained before treatment. Information from records and
from the authors' observations formed the data. The child's communicative
attempts before training were described as consisting of "combined jargon
and gestures" (p. 133). Verbally, he approximated production of six words,
using gestures and picture drawings minimally to communicate with others.
However, the child appeared to respond consistently to some environmental
sounds. Objective data were not presented for these observations. Based on
these observations, the child was started on an auditory training program. He
was trained to associate sounds with real objects such as a drum beating, bell
ringing, cutting with scissors, and so on. If the child's ability to make these
associations was assessed before training, Brookner and Murphy do not present data on the assessment. However, this behavior was not the last behavior
to be trained; in fact, the final behavior was not specified in the report. In any
case, as in most B studies, specific measurements of the behavior were not
undertaken before the initial treatment, or as the terminal behavior and
treatment changed during the course of the study. Possibly, the behaviors
trained were redefined successively on the basis of the subject's performance
as training progressed. In other words, success or failure in training dictated

the form of the behavior to be trained next. Ongoing redefinitions of terminal behaviors are frequently necessary when a client's potential for change
poses a problem, as in this study. The procedure is not unusual in B studies
and may not be critical if the purpose of the study is description. It becomes
crucial when the investigators wish to make cause and effect statements.

Treatment in the Brookner and Murphy study consisted of numerous activities over a three-year period. Specific procedures were not described in the
report, and because the program was exceedingly long and included a
number of changes, it would be unrealistic to expect detailed explanations.
In summary, words were first introduced into the auditory training program,
but when the subject failed to respond to spoken words, training shifted to
written words until the child was able to read, retain, and carry out a series of
up to six commands. When the subject had been in training about a year, a
psychological evaluation was conducted using the Bender-Gestalt Test,
Peabody Picture Vocabulary Test, WISC, and Hiskey-Nebraska Test to
measure the subject's performance on several parameters. He performed in
the educable mentally retarded range on this battery of standard tests.
Likewise, he was evaluated by the deaf education staff who recommended
that the Association Method be used in training. In this program emphasis
was placed on ability to read, say from memory, and write differently sized
units (phonemes, sequences of phonemes, and words). After a year on the
program, although it was felt that the Association Method was successful, the
subject had failed to generalize from the written material to spontaneous
speech. Therefore, a new training program of total communication was initiated in the third year of treatment. It consisted of oral speech,
speechreading, gestures, formal sign language, fingerspelling, printed word,
cursive writing, and reading. Words learned previously were used initially in
this program, and later were expanded into phrases and sentences. Owing to
a rather dramatic increase in the number of words the subject could either
sign or speak after a year of total communication training, the authors concluded, "It is obvious the total communication system brought about a
notable acceleration in his communication skills. . . . We feel it can be concluded that Johnny is responding to a total approach communication
system" (p. 136).

Presence of Scientific Components   Which of the components of the
scientific method were included in the study by Brookner and Murphy? The
components to be examined include: operational definitions, reliability,
dependent and independent variables, and control.

The behavior to be trained was designated as "oral communication
skills"; at least it appeared to be the initial target behavior. Later, it seems,
the target was changed to training a total communication system. Neither
target behavior was defined operationally with regard to various dimensions

of performance on specific tasks; neither were the exact operations to be measured for demonstrating the presence of the behavior specified. Presumably, the authors developed criteria to be met at each training step to demonstrate that the response or responses had been acquired, but if so, the criteria were not explained in the article. Lack of operational definitions can be illustrated with one example. One of the auditory training steps was designed to "expand gross sound awareness." All terms (expand, gross, sound awareness) in that purpose statement need operational definitions. An approximation to operational definitions was made in defining "gross" by listing some of the sounds and the objects associated with the sounds, such as "drum beating," "bell ringing," and so on. It was a good start on operational definitions; however, the authors did less well on the other two terms. "Expand" from what to what? How was "sound awareness" measured? The child was trained to associate recordings of the sounds with objects first and pictures of the objects later. An operational definition of the stimulus would describe how the sounds were presented, that is, at what intensity, how often, the duration of each presentation, whether they were presented free field or through headphones, and all other relevant parameters of the stimuli. Sound awareness would be defined by specifying the child's response; that is, how the child was to respond, what he was to do, how soon after the stimulus presentation he was to respond, and so on. A careful definition would indicate that the child "associated the sound with the objects." An explanation of the objective measures used to count and record the child's responses would be equally important. Finally, the authors' statement that "... the program of auditory training seemed to be progressing" (p. 133) would be supported by data on the number of stimuli presented, number of correct and incorrect responses, and meeting of a preset criterion by the child if operational definitions were used. Similar requirements for operational definitions in each training phase would be necessary if the scientific method were applied so that scientific evidence would support the authors' conclusions. Instead, Brookner and Murphy chose subjective observations as evidence of the child's progress throughout the training program (e.g., "He could identify a single noun from this core vocabulary when stimulated auditorily or visually," "He could read these patterned sentences..." (p. 134). These statements were offered without data. Subjective observations are useful in many instances, but do not fulfill the requirements demanded in a scientific investigation.

Reliability information was not presented by the authors. In the absence of reliability information the possibility of bias or idiosyncratic judgments by one person concerning the subject's performance must enter into evaluation of results.

The discussion for need of operational definitions encompasses the need for careful identification of the dependent and independent variables. The comments regarding lack of operational definitions in the Brookner and Murphy study also apply to identifying the dependent and independent variables in that study. The communicative skill or skills the subject was to acquire formed the dependent variable. In order to measure these skills they must be operationally defined. Concomitantly, the treatment program was the independent variable and each procedure in the program formed a part of the independent variable; therefore, specificity was necessary. Because neither variable was clearly defined, the effect of the treatment on communication skills was difficult to evaluate. Lack of objective data prevents statements concerning the relationship between the child's performance and the treatment.

The last component of the scientific method is important to the conclusions to be drawn from a study. This concerns the matter of designing controls to prevent interference from extraneous variables. Controls can be designed in a number of ways depending on the study format. One way in a single-subject A-B-A design is comparing occurrence of the behavior in A (baseline and after treatment) with occurrence of the behavior in B (treatment). The reversal of conditions serves to control extraneous variables present in all conditions. Thus, the occurrence of the behavior is compared between the first A and the B (before and during treatment) and again between the B and the last A (treatment and removal of treatment). If more than one treatment is administered in sequence, additional controls are needed to rule out order effects, that is, the effect of a previous treatment on the next one, and the effect of both on the third treatment, and so forth.

A treatment-only study, of course, is not designed to examine internal validity; that is, determining that behavior change is due to treatment rather than other variables. Cause and effect relationships between the treatment administered and behavioral changes requires a controlled evaluation. The B study is essentially a descriptive study, not an experimental one. This is illustrated in the Brookner and Murphy study. A comparison between performance in treatment and performance before treatment is not possible because performance was not measured before treatment, and possibly not even during treatment. Before treatment, standardized tests were administered and, although the information is interesting, the tests measured general performance or peripheral behavior (e.g., I.Q., visual perception), not the specific communication skills to be trained. Thus, occurrence of the specific responses emitted during training could not be compared to occurrence of the same responses on pretraining measures to determine if they changed when treatment was administered. The absence of comparison data prevents statements regarding the effectiveness of treatment.

Furthermore, when training is continued for a long time, three years in the Brookner and Murphy study, it is recognized that time might be a confounding variable. Time and maturation could account for the changes observed in communicative skills.

Another confounding variable may have been the educational and family environment in which the child was functioning. In these environments emphasis was placed on communicative behaviors; in fact, the foster parents participated in training. It is possible that these environmental variables were as responsible for the changes in the child's communicative skills as was the training program.

Finally, inasmuch as the total communication training followed two years of previous communicative skills training, the effect of the total communication program was confounded by the prior training. Possibly, the previous two years of communication skills training made the total communication program effective. Any other program, presented after two years of training, could have been just as effective as the total communication training.

Due to the above uncontrolled factors, statements about the effectiveness of the training programs are prohibited. Credit for changes cannot be attributed to the programs, and least of all to any one particular program.

In essence, a B study presents an interesting description, but minimal useful information. It does not allow statements regarding variables responsible for what is described any more than does a descriptive study, an A study. Yet, it is not unusual for authors and readers to draw causal inferences and to project effectiveness to training programs described in B studies, as Brookner and Murphy did. Because so many of these studies are reported in the communicative disorders literature, special care must be taken to evaluate them for scientific value. The Brookner and Murphy study was interesting, but an examination for components of the scientific method revealed that not one of the components was present. Thus, the study does not contribute information to the body of scientific knowledge, and at the most can only speculate on treatment variables. As such, it can contribute only peripherally to a scientifically based discipline. Perhaps of more interest to the content of the present text, it contributes minimal information for conducting treatment, at least for interventions derived from carefully controlled evaluation of treatment variables. Most B studies provide anecdotal and subjective evidence, rather than objectively gathered data, although they may differ in the degree to which scientific methodology is used. Nevertheless, it is obvious that a single-subject B study bears little resemblance to a single-subject experimental study. The two designs are incompatible and the purposes divergent.

The A-B Study   We come now to a design typically referred to as an A-B, or case study. Ideally an A-B study includes a well defined pretreatment assessment of the target behavior and a careful description of the treatment. Many A-only studies and B-only studies are labeled case studies, but in this text we prefer to reserve the designation for studies that allow a comparison between baseline (pretreatment) performance and performance in treatment, hence an A-B study. Certainly it is a closer approximation to an experimental single-subject design than either the A-only or B-only studies. Nonetheless, it does not qualify as an experimental study mainly because it does not include a control to rule out the effect of extraneous variables on the target behavior during the B phase. It is the careful, detailed description of the dependent and independent variables, the collection of objective data, and the use of operational definitions throughout the study that endears the well designed A-B study to researchers interested in evaluating potentially powerful treatment variables in well controlled experimental designs. An ideal case study has all of the components mentioned above, but because all case studies are not ideal, the quality varies considerably in the communicative disorders studies reported in the literature.

An example of a comprehensive A-B study of a communicative disorder is one conducted by Daniel and Guitar (1978). The study involved one 25-year-old male who had surgical anastomosis (connection) of the VIIth cranial nerve to the XIIth cranial nerve five years before the study. The subject's entire right side of the face was deficient for touch-pressure and the right side of the tongue had atrophied over the five years subsequent to the surgery. During conversational speech, the right side of the face remained passive while the left side moved expressively. Speech was normal except for a slight distortion on triple blends. The primary problem was cosmetic in that the right side of the lips and face were immobile during speech. The purpose of the study was to describe a therapy program using electromyographic (EMG) feedback for increasing coordination of facial muscular activity during speech and nonspeech events.

A detailed description of the subject's history, current performance, and physical condition was provided. Assessment consisted of testing for muscle activity with EMG. Placement of the electrodes on the subject's face and the apparatus used in evaluation and training were specified clearly. The descriptions were accompanied by drawings and illustrations to clarify exact locations. Recordings were taken from the right and left sides of the lower lip just below and parallel to the vermillion border. Other electrodes were located on specifically defined portions of the face to record bilateral muscle action potentials (MAPs). Video tapes were made of smiles early and late in therapy for measurement of lateral displacement. Additionally, measurements were made of the percentage of participation of the two sides of the mouth during production of phones. The exact locations for these measurements were described by the investigators minutely enough to allow replication.

From the initial evaluation the investigators decided that the subject might benefit from a therapy program designed to increase muscle action potentials in the lips during speech and nonspeech activities. For this training EMG feedback in the form of a tone was used to indicate to the subject how much muscle activity occurred as he exercised in training. The investigators also hypothesized that facial activity could be trained independently of tongue activity. The ultimate goal of the program was to produce symmetry in facial gestures for nonspeech and speech activities using EMG feedback.

Two nonspeech activities were developed for initial training, but before initiation of training three baseline trials with no EMG feedback were taken. During baseline the subject was allowed to use a mirror to monitor his movements, but was presented with no EMG feedback.

The two nonspeech tasks in training consisted of pressing the lips together and retracting the lips. Feedback was provided only for the right lower lip site but recordings were made from both sides. The same measurements of lip movement were made during baseline and training. At the end of training the measurements were repeated.

After baseline was obtained, the subject received ten trials with feedback and use of a mirror. The task for each of the feedback trials was specified and in summary form consisted of the following procedure. Training was begun on developing muscle activity levels for static muscle contractions, such as pressing or laterally retracting the lips. An oscillator generated a steady tone that was amplified by a loudspeaker in the soundproofed IAC booth where the subject sat. When the subject's MAPs exceeded a selected threshold level, the oscillator-generated tone increased in frequency proportional to the MAP increase. In this way the client could monitor his changing MAP levels by listening to the frequency of the tone as he contracted and relaxed his muscles.

His task was to keep the tone above the center frequency for 5 seconds. To progress to the next training step the subject had to complete 10 consecutive successful trials. In each step more muscle activity was required to keep the tone above the center frequency for 5 seconds. By decreasing amplifier gain, an increase in muscle activity was required to activate the oscillator and the signal. This forced the subject to produce greater muscle activity at each progressive step. In addition to the EMG feedback and the mirror in training, the subject was instructed to keep the tongue relaxed and the face symmetrical. He was also provided with a bite block to hold between the teeth to keep lip movement independent of jaw movement. When the nonspeech MAPs reached criterion levels, speech training was initiated. The procedures for this training were explained by the authors as explicitly as the nonspeech training. In the final stages of training the subject was producing conversational speech, was not allowed to use a mirror, and feedback was provided only occasionally by verbal reminders from a speech-language pathologist.

Results were presented graphically for the pressing, retraction, eversion, and lip-lifting activities. Levels of lower-lip muscular activity in microvolts across training sessions were presented in a figure on training data. In addition, tables of pretraining and posttraining measures of the percentage of participation of the two sides of the lips during phone production were included in the results section of the report. The findings included: 1) increases in muscular activity in the lower lip, 2) lack of changes in the upper lip during lip lifting, 3) independence of the facial muscle activity from conscious tongue contractions, and 4) evidence that the feedback training was effective.

In discussing the results, the authors were careful to explain that the changes cannot be attributed solely to the EMG feedback procedure because other variables were present during treatment. They point out possible reasons why the feedback might have been responsible, but recognize the tentative nature of this conclusion.

Presence of Scientific Components   A comparison of the three studies discussed in this section (the A-only, the B-only, and the A-B) should make it eminently clear that the A-B study includes more of the components of the scientific method than the other two. With a few qualifications, the Daniel and Guitar study includes operational definitions, identification of dependent and independent variables, and reliability. Only the control component is lacking completely. The study has other components meeting the requirements of an experimental design. The basic components will be addressed in this section, but when appropriate, other components contributing to a good design will be pointed out.

It is apparent that Daniel and Guitar defined most of the relevant parameters operationally, enabling them to use objective measures in examining events occurring before and during intervention. To begin with, their definitions of the dependent and independent variables attest to use of operational definitions. Although dependent and independent variables are often reserved for use in describing only experimental studies, they form the central components of any study in which treatment is administered with the expectation that a behavioral change will result, and it is in this light they are discussed. The dependent variable was defined as changes in amount of muscle activity in the right lip during nonspeech and speech exercises, whereas the independent variable was defined as EMG feedback on lip movement. In order to obtain objective data on these variables, lip movement was defined so that it could be directly measured instrumentally. Reliance was not placed on subjective perceptual judgments of humans. Measurements from several places around the lips were obtained to gain a comprehensive record of the movement. Thus, for example, lip pressing and lip retracting were defined as muscle activity measured via electrodes placed on or near the muscles involved during lip pressing and retracting. Likewise, the independent variable, EMG feedback, was defined by describing precisely how the oscillator functioned to provide feedback. (More will be said about the independent variable later.)

Not only were operational definitions used in identifying the dependent and independent variables, the training procedures were operationally defined by specifying clearly what occurred in each session. The procedures were specified with regard to: 1) what constituted a trial, 2) the number of trials per step, 3) criterion level to be reached at each step, and 4) how changes in the independent variable were programmed. Needless to say, not all aspects of the training program were equally clearly defined, but operational definitions accompanied the majority of them.

Reliability is another component of the scientific method. Measurement of the EMG records traced on graph paper during operation of the EMG was specified by the investigators. They noted that 10% of the training trials were selected for remeasurement for reliability determination. The standard error of measurement was computed and reported. Similarly, measurements for percentage of participation of the two sides of the mouth in phone production as recorded on videotapes were repeated for reliability. It is appropriate to obtain reliability in any measure involving human judgment. Although in the Daniel and Guitar study instruments were used to obtain direct and objective measurements, humans were required to analyze the tracings from the instruments. The need to have humans analyze the records made reliability information necessary. Hopefully, two different individuals were involved in the two measures so that independent judgments were obtained.

The next two components to be discussed are the dependent and independent variables. Operational definitions of both have already been established. The independent variable requires further discussion because the investigators' definition was incomplete. The authors indicated that the EMG feedback was the independent variable. In reality, the treatment consisted of several variables because it included: 1) EMG feedback, 2) use of a mirror by the subject to observe lip movement, 3) consistently administered instructions to the subject about what he should be doing, and 4) a bite block to insure independence of lip and jaw movement. In baseline the subject was allowed to use the mirror, so that particular variable could have been ruled out as a confounding variable because it was a constant in both conditions (i.e., baseline and training). The instructions and bite block, however, were not present during baseline measurement. They were introduced in training when the EMG feedback was introduced. Therefore, the independent variable consisted of three treatments in addition to the mirror, and the effect of any one variable could not be evaluated. Of the four variables in treatment (EMG feedback, mirror, instructions, and bite block), only the EMG feedback was specified and operationally defined.

We come now to the final component, control. And this, of course, is what distinguishes a case study of a single subject from a single-subject experimental study. Because the design has only a baseline and treatment phase, the effect of other variables during treatment cannot be ruled out. It is possible, for example, in the Daniel and Guitar study that the subject had started spontaneously to recover lip movement at the same time training was introduced, or that the subject was involved in another kind of training outside the therapy setting that was responsible for the increased muscle movement seen in training, or that other unidentified variables were influencing the subject's performance. To demonstrate the effect of the independent variable it is necessary to control for such extraneous variables.

An A-B study is not designed to control for these extraneous variables and that is not the purpose of an A-B study. Daniel and Guitar recognized the possible confounding and discussed the tentative nature of conclusions concerning the effectiveness of EMG feedback. They might have added to that the tentative nature of any conclusions that the training was responsible for increased muscle movement, because the effectiveness of the treatment was not evaluated properly.

Keeping in mind that the Daniel and Guitar study had shortcomings, it is still possible to rate it as an example of a nearly ideal A-B study. With a few modifications it could be redesigned as an A-B-A within-subject experimental study. The A-B-A and A-B-A-B single-subject designs are described in Chapter 2.

SUMMARY

All experimental studies include the basic components of the scientific method: operational definitions, reliability, dependent and independent variables, and control. In group designs control is provided by dividing the subjects into control and experimental groups. Treatment is administered only to the experimental group. In the within-subject design, control is provided by administering all experimental conditions to the subjects. Thus, the rationale for the two research methodologies differs. To design a proper single-subject experimental study it is necessary to comprehend the difference in rationale.

Many single-subject studies are descriptive, not experimental, in nature. Included in this group are the A-only study, the B-only study, and the A-B study. The A-B case study usually includes the greatest number of scientific components; hence, it approximates the experimental within-subject design used to evaluate treatment variables in a controlled manner. It is necessary to keep in mind, however, that the A-only, B-only, and A-B designs allow restricted statements concerning the effectiveness of proposed and applied treatment variables.

Withdrawal and Reversal Designs

2

A primary goal of an applied behavioral analysis is to provide a convincing demonstration of experimental control over the occurrence and nonoccurrence of target behaviors. In contrast to the "quasi-experimental" designs (Campbell and Stanley, 1966) discussed in the previous chapter, the A-B-A design provides a degree of control that allows an assessment of cause and effect relationships between experimental variables and the behaviors to which they are applied. The purpose of this chapter is to discuss factors relevant to the evaluation and implementation of single-subject reversal designs. However, because single-subject research strategies represent a distinct departure from the traditional group study approach to communicative disorders research, it is necessary to begin this discussion with several introductory remarks.

The intrasubject designs considered in this text have been classified as *time-series* designs. Simply stated, this approach involves the continuous measurement of a dependent variable over an extended period of time and monitoring the effects of an independent variable (e.g., treatment) on the series of measurements. Thus, continuous data collection is an important aspect of within-subject research designs. Moreover, direct observation of a target behavior during periods when treatment is present and when it is not may reveal whether treatment is responsible for alterations in that behavior. As previously noted, there are two principal phases of a within-subject study, an *A,* or baseline phase, and a *B,* or treatment phase. Intervention is judged to be effective if changes in the behavior co-occur with the presentation and removal of treatment during these phases.

In addition to being a "time-series" analysis, it is important to note that the subject "serves as his own control" in experimental single-subject studies. In the A-B-A and other within-subject designs to be discussed, appropriate experimental control is possible, in part, because each subject participates in all experimental conditions. Because potentially confounding factors are likely present throughout each phase, the subject is equally exposed to extraneous influences during both treatment and nontreatment conditions. Similarly, any uncontrolled variables powerful enough to effect a change in behavior would be expected to do so in all of the experimental phases. Therefore, if behavioral change corresponds with the manipulation of the treatment variable but never occurs during nontreatment phases, one can conclude that the influence of confounding variables was negligible. Importantly, this presupposes that all experimental conditions other than treatment have been held constant across phases. Otherwise, the effect of treatment cannot be separated from the effect of the nontreatment variables that were allowed to vary.

It was previously noted that the group study approach to treatment research relies on a statistical comparison between the mean performance of experimental and control groups to assess treatment effectiveness. In contrast, the results of single-case experimental designs are generally presented on a graph and direct visual inspection of an individual's performance provides the primary method of data analysis. There are several advantages to this method of data analysis. First, because raw data are plotted and analyzed during each phase of a study, the experimenter is kept in close contact with his results and is in a position to know if the data are conforming to preexperimental expectations. This allows appropriate modifications in the study protocol as problems arise and provides a considerable degree of experimental flexibility. In addition, graphing of raw data permits other members of the scientific community to assess independently the power of obtained results. Finally, when the criterion for acceptance of data is a marked effect evident from visual inspection, variables having a weak treatment effect will be teased out and powerful variables will be retained and further explored.

THE A-B-A WITHDRAWAL DESIGN

It can be seen that a firm grasp of the methods of graphing and visual inspection of data is essential to understanding single-subject research strategies. Therefore, it will be necessary to review briefly the basic form of data presentation utilized in within-subject studies. The example that follows is also used to introduce the A-B-A withdrawal design.

Although numerous types and combinations of graphs have been used to present data from single case experimental designs, the most common is the line graph. Figure 1 presents an idealized line graph from an A-B-A withdrawal design. Each of the components of the graph is explained and subsequently discussed in the context of a hypothetical example of a withdrawal design.

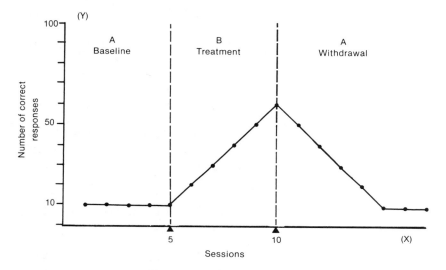

Figure 1. Results of a hypothetical study depicting the experimental phases of an A-B-A withdrawal design.

The solid horizontal and vertical lines on the graph represent the abscissa (X axis) and the ordinate (Y axis), respectively. The dependent variable, the behavior being studied, is often measured in rate, frequency, or percent of change that occurs and is plotted along the ordinate. In the Daniel and Guitar (1978) study discussed in the previous chapter, for example, the dependent variable was the amount of labial muscle activity and was presented in microvolts along this axis. Time is generally plotted along the abscissa in single-subject research. In the above example, the change in muscular activity was measured across the number of sessions in which training occurred.

The three phases of an A-B-A design depicted in the figure are separated by vertical lines and each is designated as a baseline (A) or treatment (B) condition. The initial A or baseline phase consists of a series of observations of the dependent variable before the initiation of treatment. The importance of adequate baseline measurement in within-subject research cannot be overstated, as it serves as the basis of comparison for evaluating the effectiveness of treatment. Moreover, an adequate comparison of the rate or frequency of behavior during baseline and treatment phases is only possible when a stable rate of baseline responding is obtained. The presence of a stable baseline, for example, rules out maturation or repeated testing as possible confounding variables, because any influences of these factors on behavior would be exhibited by a trend toward improvement during baseline. If improvement is noted in baseline performance and it continues after treatment is applied, one does not know whether the behavioral change is due to intervention, or if it is simply a continuation of the trend observed during baseline. Similarly, a highly variable baseline, in which there is alternating improvement and deterioration in performance, prohibits an assessment of the efficacy of treatment. This is particularly true when data from the treatment phase are also variable and overlap in level with the baseline phase. The effect of treatment is primarily seen as a marked vertical change in level of the data line once intervention has begun and variability tends to obscure such changes. The data display during the baseline phase of the figure represents a stable base rate of responding. Note that there is no change in the slope of the line that might indicate a trend toward improvement.

The "B" phase shown in the figure represents the treatment portion of the study. A vertical alteration in the data during this phase is indicative of improvement. In the present example, the number of occurrences of the behavior depicted in the figure gradually increases throughout the treatment phase. Assuming that all factors from the baseline phase were held constant, the marked improvement in performance at the initiation of treatment provides evidence of experimental control and treatment effectiveness (first arrow). This evidence alone, however, is not conclusive. As noted in the discussion of the A-B design, one cannot rule out alternate explanations that may account for improvement in behavior on the basis of a single baseline-treatment comparison. The addition of a withdrawal phase (A) provides the additional experimental control needed. If treatment was powerful enough to alter the subject's behavior during the intervention phase, removal of the experimental contingencies during the withdrawal phase should result in an extinction of the newly acquired behavior. That is, improvement should be reversed toward baseline if treatment is withdrawn. The second arrow in the figure marks the beginning of the withdrawal phase of the study. It can be seen that a decrease in the behavior corresponded with the removal of treatment and continued throughout the withdrawal phase. Together with the first evidence of experimental control, marked improvement in performance when treatment was introduced, this subsequent decrease in occurrence of the behavior when treatment is withdrawn would establish sufficient experimental control to conclude that the treatment was responsible for the observed change in behavior.

Having briefly discussed the logic of the withdrawal design, it may be instructive to reexamine the figure within the context of a hypothetical A-B-A study. A single-subject withdrawal design could, for example, be used to examine the relationship between the "digital pressure" technique and increased length of phonation for esophageal speakers. A duration of phonation of ≥ 2 seconds is considered to be sufficient for intelligible esophageal speech. Therefore, it may be important to explore techniques that appear to increase length and consistency of phonation for alaryngeal patients. One technique, the use of digital neck pressure, reportedly permits acceptable phonation in patients who have difficulty trapping or expelling sufficient air to produce esophageal speech.

If an A-B-A study was designed to explore the effectiveness of this approach to esophageal speech training, the dependent variable in the study could be duration of vowel phonation. Alternately, the independent variable could be a treatment package that included specific clinician instruction and digital compression on the subject's neck at the level of the sound source. During the baseline (A) phase the subject would be asked to phonate the vowel /a/ upon command. Duration of vowel phonation would be carefully timed using a voice-operated relay and an electrical timer. Correct responses would be defined as vowels that were produced for ≥ 2 seconds and all other responses would be scored incorrect. No instructions would be provided about the use of digital pressure during baseline; the duration of vowel phonation would simply be monitored. Once a stable rate of responding was attained during baseline, the treatment phase (B) would begin. During this phase the subject would be instructed about the use of digital pressure and he would apply appropriate pressure at a selected site on his neck in attempting to increase the length of vowel phonation. All other factors would be held constant and the experimenter would continue to measure duration of phonation to determine the effect of treatment. Upon reaching a predetermined performance criterion, the withdrawal phase (A) of the study would be implemented. This would involve the removal of treatment and reinstatement of the baseline phase conditions.

If we were to use Figure 1 to represent the results of this study, the number of correct vowel productions would be plotted along the ordinate and the number of sessions would be presented along the abscissa. Inspection of the graph would reveal that the subject consistently produced 10 correct responses during each of the baseline sessions and a stable baseline would have been obtained. The treatment (B) condition of this study would have begun after session five. It is apparent from the figure that improvement in the subject's ability to phonate on command for the specified duration co-occurred with the initiation of treatment and continued throughout the intervention phase. During the withdrawal phase (A) of the study the instruction-digital pressure treatment package would have been withdrawn. This manipulation corresponds to the rapid deterioration in performance evident throughout the withdrawal phase of the figure. Based on the rapid increase in the number of correct vowel phonations during the treatment phase and the reversal of performance after the removal of treatment, one might conclude that the hypothetical treatment was successful.

Although the A-B-A design has not been used to its fullest extent by researchers in speech pathology and related fields, it provides a powerful means of investigating treatment effectiveness. Furthermore, a complete understanding of this design is prerequisite to consideration of more sophisticated withdrawal designs. Therefore, an example of this design from the communicative disorders literature is presented and discussed in the section that follows.

Investigators in stuttering were among the first within the field of communicative disorders to recognize the power and elegance of single-case methodologies. An early study by Martin and Siegel (1966), for example, examined the effects of response-contingent positive and negative verbal feedback on the rate of dysfluency produced by two adult male stutterers. The experimental setting for the study consisted of a control room, from which the experimenter delivered verbal consequation and tallied the number of dysfluencies produced, and an experimental room. The experimental task required the subject to read a prose passage throughout each of the eight sessions. All subject responses were tape recorded, and a hand-held switch automatically tallied the number of stuttering moments produced during each 2–minute period of each session. The first session and the first few minutes of each subsequent session were dedicated to baseline testing. During baseline (A) the subject was asked to read continuously, but no instructions or feedback were provided. A baseline stability criterion was set that permitted a predetermined rate of variability in the frequency of stuttering produced during three consecutive 2–minute periods of reading. An additional stability criterion required that, for any given session, the subject had to have read for a minimum of 10 minutes before meeting an acceptable level of stability. The first treatment (B) phase began during the second experimental session after a stable base rate had been demonstrated during the first 10 minutes of the session.

Treatment consisted of instructions, to "...read very carefully. Don't worry about keeping the sentence going, just say each word fluently" (Martin and Siegel, 1966, p. 469). Contingent delivery of "not good" was presented after each moment of stuttering and "good" was presented after each 30 seconds of fluency. The treatment phase lasted for 30 minutes and was followed by a withdrawal (A) phase. The withdrawal phase consisted of removal of instructions and verbal contingencies and reinstatement of baseline conditions.

The results of this study are depicted in Figure 2 for subject "N" for a single experimental session. The dependent variable, number of dysfluencies produced during 2–minute periods, is plotted on the ordinate and duration

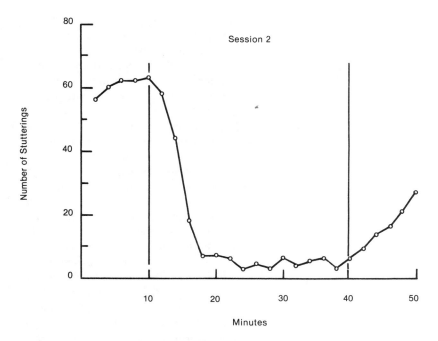

Figure 2. Number of stutterings emitted by subject N every 2 minutes during session 2 (50 minutes). Base rate for first 10 minutes. Instructions given, "not good" delivered contingent upon each stuttering and "good" delivered contingent upon each 30 seconds of fluency for next 30 minutes. No stimuli delivered for last 10 minutes. (From Martin and Siegel, 1966, p. 470. Copyright (1966) by the American Speech and Hearing Association. Reproduced with permission).

of the experimental session is plotted along the abscissa. Examination of the figure reveals that the number of dysfluencies emitted during each 2–minute baseline period was approximately 60. The small range of variability between the baseline data points and absence of improved performance is indicative of a stable baseline. Further examination of the graph reveals that the number of dysfluencies began to decrease at the beginning of the treatment phase, and a rapid improvement was evident during the first 8 minutes of intervention. The improvement leveled off at approximately five dysfluencies per 2–minute period and subsequently continued at this level for the remainder of the treatment condition. Thus, the co-occurrence of a marked improvement in fluency and the application of treatment provide partial support for the effectiveness of the training package. Data from the withdrawal (A) phase of the study are presented for the final 10 minutes of the session. Visual inspection of the graph reveals that there was a steady increase in the number of stuttering moments. In conjunction with the improvement seen during the intervention phase, these results support the conclusion that the treatment package and change in rate of stuttering behavior were functionally related. That is, the behavior change appears to have been a result of treatment. Martin and Siegel (1966) concluded that ''. . . punishing stuttering and reinforcing fluency proved to be an effective means of reducing stuttering and increasing fluency'' (p. 474).

Although inspection of Figure 2 appears to support the conclusion that treatment was effective, it is important to consider reasonable alternative explanations and possible confounding variables when evaluating the results of any study. Data that are convincing through visual assessment are only conclusive when appropriate experimental controls have been utilized throughout each phase of the study. In the present study, for example, instructions were provided during the treatment phase that were not presented during the baseline and withdrawal phases, an apparent violation of the ''one variable rule'' (Hersen and Barlow, 1976). This rule states that only one variable should be manipulated when proceeding from one experimental phase to the next. When more than one factor is altered between phases, it is not possible to determine the effect of any single variable on subject's performance (see Interaction Designs, p. 194). Martin and Siegel's (1966) conclusion that verbal contingencies were solely responsible for changes in fluency must, therefore, be qualified because instructions may also have influenced the obtained results.[1] The experimenter's instructions may have interacted with praise and admonishment and accounted for all, or perhaps none of the observed effect.

A second factor that should be considered is the length of experimental phases in this study. From an examination of Figure 2, it is evident that the treatment phase is considerably longer than the baseline and withdrawal phases. Strictly speaking, this makes baseline / treatment comparisons problematic because the relatively longer duration of the treatment phase presents a greater opportunity for confounding variables to affect the rate of stuttering during this phase as compared to the baseline or withdrawal phase. As Hersen and Barlow (1976) note, each phase should contain a relatively equal number of observations whenever possible.

Ultimately, the influence of unequal experimental phases must be assessed along with the amount of experimental control exercised throughout the study. In the present example, the experimental design could have been modified so that equal phases would have been possible throughout the

---

[1]Martin and Siegel (1966) acknowledged the possible influence of instructions and attempted to examine this variable. Unfortunately, their analysis was limited to an A-B study and was therefore inconclusive.

study. In the vast majority of communicative disorders treatment research, however, practical limitations prevent the use of equivalent phases and a performance criterion is usually set to determine the length of the treatment phase. Given that individual subject's rate of learning may vary considerably, it is often not feasible to closely regulate the length of a treatment phase. Although not ideal, the use of unequal experimental phases is not a major limitation to the use of within-subject designs in communicative disorders studies when an unambiguous treatment effect has been demonstrated.

Violations of the one-variable rule, unequal length of experimental phases and other potential confounds must be considered when experimental results are being evaluated. Although visual-graphic analysis serves as the primary means of evaluating single-subject data, visual analysis must be accompanied by a critical assessment of factors that may compromise results and conclusions. Criteria for evaluating the results of within-subject studies are thoroughly discussed in Chapter 4.

Although the A-B-A withdrawal is one of the most basic single-case experimental designs, it has been used infrequently by investigators in the area of communicative disorders. This may, in part, be due to the belated recognition of within-subject research strategies in the allied health fields and the concomitant increase in the level of sophistication of the applied behavior analysis methodologies in recent years. Furthermore, objections raised about the appropriateness of withdrawal designs for specific clinical populations may have contributed to the infrequent use of this design. Starkweather (1971), for example, argued against the use of the A-B-A design in stuttering experimentation and suggested the use of several alternative designs. And Davis (1978) has questioned the usefulness of withdrawal designs for studying aphasic language impairments. Despite these objections, withdrawal and reversal designs have been fruitfully applied with both populations (Kearns and Salmon, in press; Costello and Hurst, 1981).

The limited use of withdrawal designs to study communicatively impaired patients may also be related to the assumption that this experimental methodology is ethically objectionable. Proponents of this view argue that withholding treatment from a subject in an attempt to demonstrate experimental control involves depriving a subject of needed treatment. This position, however, is based on the tenuous assumption that the treatment withheld from a subject would be of benefit to him. The illogic of this assumption is apparent when it is recalled that the primary purpose of using withdrawal and other single-subject designs is to determine whether a given treatment is effective for modifying behavior. Thus, by providing a method for examining the validity of a given treatment, a successful series of studies that uses withdrawal methodologies may help professionals avoid the ethically questionable practice of using unproven treatment procedures.

A practical limitation of withdrawal and reversal designs related to the above ethical considerations is the possibility of staff resistance to their implementation (Hersen and Barlow, 1976). Clinicians and others not fully informed of the rationale behind the experimental removal of apparently successful treatment may not fully cooperate in carrying out a study protocol. This problem may be more acute in settings such as nursing homes and institutions in which the professional staff have not received specialized training. Moreover, reluctance to adopt single-case withdrawal designs may be especially evident when an A-B-A design is being used because such studies are terminated after subject's performance has been reversed to the pretreatment level of functioning. This is a serious limitation of the A-B-A design because such studies are generally undertaken to evaluate the effectiveness of a training procedure or program that may have remedial potential. One might reasonably question the rationale for terminating a study after a withdrawal phase when results indicate that reinstatement of treatment may be beneficial to a given subject. Practical problems such as subject attrition may, of course, prevent the reinstatement of treatment after experimental control has been demonstrated. Whenever possible, however, studies should not be terminated after a withdrawal or reversal phase. Several extensions of the basic A-B-A design that end after a treatment rather than a reversal phase are considered in the following section.

THE B-A-B WITHDRAWAL DESIGN

Experimental control is possible using the A-B-A withdrawal design because the effect of both the application and removal of an independent variable can be observed within each subject. Each experimental phase provides data from which the experimenter can predict what the level of performance is likely to be during subsequent phases if the experimental contingencies remained unchanged (Kazdin, 1977b). Thus, if a stable rate of behavior is evident during a baseline phase one would predict that intervention should accelerate or decelerate the rate of responding. Assuming that this prediction was correct and improvement was evident, the results of the treatment phase would lead one to predict that withdrawal of the experimental contingencies would result in a deterioration in performance and a return to the baseline level of responding. Experimental control is demonstrated when changes in performance correspond with the predicted outcome each time a treatment variable is applied or withdrawn. The A-B-A design permits such predictions, in part, because a no-treatment, treatment, no-treatment (withdrawal) sequence is followed. Other permutations of the A-B-A design in which treatment and no-treatment conditions alternate in consecutive phases also provide a convincing means of demonstrating experimental control and one of these, the B-A-B withdrawal, is considered in the following discussion.

As indicated by its name, the B-A-B design begins with a treatment (B) rather than a baseline phase. After a stable rate of responding has been obtained at a specified criterion level, intervention is withdrawn (A) to determine if treatment had been responsible for maintaining the stable rate obtained during the initial treatment phase. Intervention is then reinstated (B) during the final experimental phase. As in the A-B-A and other withdrawal or reversal designs, each phase of the B-A-B withdrawal is used as a basis for comparing the effects of experimental manipulations on adjacent phases. Moreover, performance in each phase permits a prediction of expected outcome for subsequent experimental conditions. A hypothetical example of this design may prove instructive, because this design has seldom been employed in the communicative disorders literature.

The process of teacher or clinical supervision in the fields of speech pathology, audiology, deaf education, and learning disabilities has seldom been experimentally investigated and the efficacy of many techniques used to train clinicians and teachers has yet to be documented. However, withdrawal and reversal designs may be useful for providing a data base in this area. The B-A-B withdrawal design could, for example, be used to investigate the effects of supervisor feedback on clinical performance. Let us assume that a supervisor is overseeing a student's management of the language deficiencies of an adult head trauma victim. The "language of confusion" apparent in such patients is often characterized by irrelevant and confabulatory responses, particularly in open-ended situations (Wertz, 1978). Therefore, one clinical goal that might be established for such a patient is reduction in the number of irrelevant or confabulatory verbal responses. For the purposes of our hypothetical example, let us assume that a student-clinician presents a series of sequentially related stimulus pictures and the patient's task is to describe verbally each activity in the sequence. Let us further assume that during the course of treatment the clinician's supervisor observes that the clinician frequently engages in off-task discussion with the patient after confabulatory or irrelevant patient response. As a result of this observation the supervisor could implement a program consisting of verbal feedback and praise in an attempt to reduce the amount of off-task behavior exhibited by the clinician. The B-A-B withdrawal design could be used by the supervisor to determine the effectiveness of his or her attempts to modify the clinician's behavior. The independent variable in such a hypothetical study would be the supervisor-imposed training program (verbal praise and feedback) and the dependent variable would be the number of off-task clinician responses.

During the initial phase (B) of the investigation the supervisor would observe and listen to the treatment sessions behind a one-way mirror, while the clinician and the patient were engaged in the verbal sequencing task described previously. Although the clinician would be able to listen to the supervisor's feedback through an audio loop system, the patient would not hear the supervisor. In addition, the supervisor would not be seen by the clinician or the patient. Corrective feedback would be provided contingent upon off-task clinician behavior and on-task clinician behavior would be praised. Once a stable rate of responding had been established, verbal feedback and consequation would be removed during a withdrawal (A) phase. If the program had been effective in modifying the clinician's behavior, removal of the training package should result in a deterioration in performance. That is, the number of off-task behaviors would likely increase once the contingencies were removed. The final phase of the study, the retraining (B) phase, would be implemented once a high, stable rate of off-task responding was established through the withdrawal procedures. This phase would be essentially equivalent to the initial training phase. The study would be terminated after improvement in the clinician's performance had been stabilized at a predetermined criterion level.

As the above example demonstrates, the B-A-B design may provide a useful strategy for examining clinical research issues in communicative disorders. As compared to A-B-A withdrawal and reversal designs, the B-A-B has one major advantage. Specifically, a subject is terminated from a B-A-B study at the end of a treatment phase, thereby circumventing the objectionable practice of dismissing a subject after a withdrawal of treatment. There is also, however, a serious limitation of B-A-B designs that is worthy of comment. Unlike the A-B-A design, the B-A-B does not begin with a baseline phase and consequently there is no basis for comparing treatment effects with the natural frequency of occurrence of the target behavior. Thus, the amount of improvement that occurs during the initial intervention phase of a B-A-B study is difficult to assess. Furthermore, the influence of extraneous variables that might have affected the initial acquisition of a target behavior cannot always be determined when a B-A-B design is implemented. A B-A-B design initiated after a behavior has been acquired only reveals whether the treatment under investigation is controlling a subject's behavior. It is possible, however, that other factors may have been in effect when the behavior was acquired but are no longer in effect. Moreover, such factors may have been critical during the acquisition of a target response but treatment alone may be sufficient to maintain performance after the extraneous variables are no longer present.

As we have seen, both the A-B-A and B-A-B withdrawal designs have strengths and limitations that merit careful consideration. Many of the limitations of the designs are, however, overcome by using an A-B-A-B design.

THE A-B-A-B WITHDRAWAL DESIGN

The A-B-A-B design is one of the most powerful single-case experimental designs available (Leitenberg, 1973). Procedurally, the design consists of a basic A-B-A approach extended by the addition of a final treatment phase. This is an important modification because it overcomes the major limitation of the A-B-A design by ending with a treatment rather than a no-treatment phase. The A-B-A-B is likely to be more acceptable to clinicians and administrators because it circumvents objections to terminating a study during a reversal phase. In addition, this design is preferable to the B-A-B design because the initial baseline phase provides information concerning the natural frequency of occurrence of a target behavior before intervention.

Figure 3 presents an idealized graph of data from an A-B-A-B design. Note the similarities between the components and data presented in this figure and those presented in the A-B-A design in Figure 1.

Experimental control is demonstrated with the A-B-A-B design in the same manner previously discussed for its basic counterpart. That is, if changes in the rate of the target behavior co-occur with application and removal of treatment, it is highly probable that the change was functionally related to treatment. The three arrows below the abscissa designate places on the graph where initiation or removal of treatment corresponded with a change in behavior. It can be seen that improvement in performance occurred at the beginning of the initial treatment phase (first arrow) and continued throughout this phase. The subsequent withdrawal of treatment is marked by the second arrow. Removal of the hypothetical treatment resulted in a decrease in the rate of behavior produced during this phase. To this point, the design is essentially an A-B-A design and sufficient experimental control

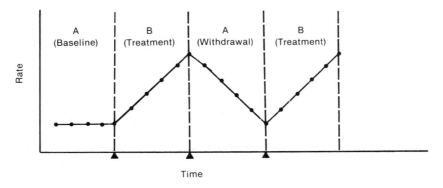

Figure 3. Results of a hypothetical study depicting the experimental phases of an A-B-A-B withdrawal design.

could have been shown. However, reinstatement of treatment during the final phase of the study (third arrow) and the associated replication of the training effect provides additional evidence that the behavior was a result of manipulation of the therapeutic variable. Taken together, the correspondence between manipulation of a treatment and change in behavior at three separate periods within the same subject in an A-B-A-B design provides convincing evidence that treatment was effective in controlling the target behavior. The following example demonstrates the usefulness of the A-B-A-B design.

Marked anterior tongue protrusion during speech or swallowing has been found in association with dental malocclusion and articulatory disorders, and it is generally considered to be deviant when it persists beyond the preschool years. Yet very little data exist with regard to remedial measures to correct this problem and tongue thrust therapy has remained a controversial topic in the communicative disorders literature. Thompson, Iwata, and Poynter (1979), however, utilized an A-B-A-B withdrawal design to study the effects of "differential reinforcement and punishment" on pathological tongue thrust in a spastic cerebral palsied child.

The subject of this study was a 10–year-old profoundly retarded cerebral palsied child. In addition to his intellectual and motoric deficits, a significant hearing loss and visual impairment were also reported. The study was conducted during daily school lunch periods and sessions varied from 10 to 30 minutes in duration. At the beginning of each session the subject was carefully secured into the same seating position to ensure that postural variability did not affect his performance. During the baseline (A) phase, small spoonfuls of food were presented to the subject whenever his mouth was empty, regardless of tongue position. A 10–second interval recording system was used to record the percentage of occurrence of tongue protrusion, food expulsion, and chewing throughout the study. The procedures followed during the treatment phase (B) of the study paralleled those from the baseline phase, except the food was presented contingent on the subject's having his tongue inside his mouth. A contingent pushback procedure was also implemented. This involved gently pushing the subject's tongue back into his mouth with a spoon each time it protruded past the middle of his lower lip. The interval scoring system continued during this phase and data were also collected on the contingent pushback procedure. The withdrawal phase (A) of the study consisted of a return to baseline. That is, the contingencies present during the treatment phase were removed and the dependent behaviors were again simply monitored. The terminal phase (B) of the study consisted of a reinstatement of the contingent feeding and pushback procedure. Although a follow-up phase and social validation procedures were also incorporated into this study, the present discussion will be restricted to the A-B-A-B phases of the withdrawal design. Furthermore, only the results for tongue thrusting (protrusion) will be considered.

The results of the study are presented in Figure 4. Examination of Figure 4 reveals that tongue thrusting occurred during a high proportion of the

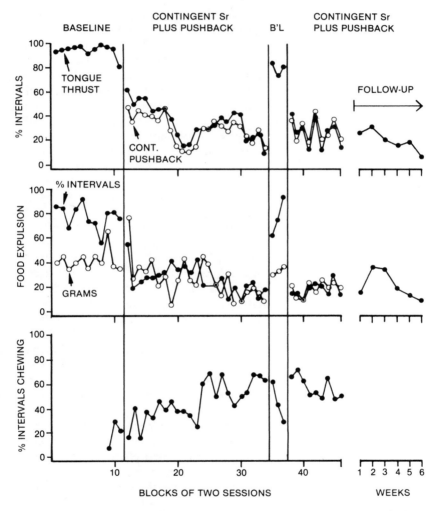

Figure 4. Percentage intervals of tongue out (target behavior) and contingent pushback (experimenter behavior) across experimental conditions. Also shown are data on food expulsion (both percentage intervals and grams) and chewing (percentage intervals). (From Thompson, Jr. et al. 1979, p. 330. Copyright by Society for the Experimental Analysis of Behavior, Inc. Reproduced with permission).

baseline intervals. In fact, the subject's tongue was protruded for an average of approximately 95 % of the intervals during this phase. It should be noted, however, that there was a slight trend toward improvement during the last few baseline data points. This is particularly evident for the last baseline interval in which tongue thrusting decreased to approximately 80 %. After introduction of the second phase, the percentage of intervals in which thrusting occurred was reduced to an average of 37 % and the target behavior was emitted in fewer than 20 % by the end of this phase. The subsequent return to baseline (A) essentially replicated the results of the initial baseline phase. An immediate and dramatic increase in tongue protrusion followed the withdrawal of treatment. Similarly, reapplication of treatment during the final phase (B) resulted in a decrease in thrusting, which paralleled that event during the first treatment phase. Based on these results, Thompson, et al. (1979) concluded that "procedures based on operant conditioning principles can effectively control observable components of tongue thrust" (p. 331).

Initial visual inspection of the data from this withdrawal design would seem to support the authors' overall conclusion that treatment was effective in controlling tongue thrusting. The authors provided appropriate definitions of the relevant behaviors and the experimental procedures were, generally, well described. In addition, inter- and intra-judge reliability measures were, for the most part, within an acceptable range. As previously noted, however, there was a tendency toward improvement at the end of the baseline phase which may have continued without the treatment phase, thereby confounding the results of the study. In addition, "myofunctional" therapy was held before each experimental session during the study, and the effect of this concurrent training on the subject's performance cannot be determined.

In the above example, and in the previous example for the A-B-A design, treatment variables were simply removed during the withdrawal phase in an attempt to demonstrate experimental control and examine treatment effectiveness. A variation of this procedure may also be implemented when an investigator is particularly interested in comparing the effects of contingent and noncontingent reinforcement or when target behaviors are produced at a negligible level in the absence of reinforcement (Sulzer-Azaroff and Mayer, 1977; Kazdin, 1977b). This variation involves the presentation of noncontingent reinforcement during the withdrawal phase rather than the total removal of all experimental events. This procedure has the advantage of having reinforcers available throughout the withdrawal phase of an experiment and this may help to maintain attention and responding in subjects who are hyperactive or inattentive.

As previously noted, the A-B-A-B withdrawal design overcomes the major weakness of the A-B-A design because the design ends after a treatment phase. Consequently, subjects are terminated from a study at a time when they have gained maximally from the treatment under study. An additional benefit derived from reinstating treatment during the final phase of the A-B-A-B sequence is that both no-treatment (A) and treatment conditions (B) are replicated within the same subject. The additional replication within this design strengthens the conclusions that can be reached by the investigator because the effect of experimentally manipulating the independent variable can be observed three times with this design (see arrows in Figure 3). Thus, the A-B-A-B is more powerful than its A-B-A counterpart in which the effect of only two experimental manipulations can be observed (see arrows in Figure 1).

Although addition of the final phase in the A-B-A-B design will increase the duration of the study, the benefits gained seemed to far outweigh the inconvenience and associated costs. When time is a critical factor or when removal of experimental contingencies is not expected to result in a return to baseline, an A-B-A-B reversal design may be the design of choice. This and other reversal designs will be considered in the next section.

THE A-B-A REVERSAL DESIGN

The experimental logic of withdrawal and reversal designs is identical and until recently, the two designs have not often been distinguished (Leitenberg, 1973; Hersen and Barlow, 1976). In each group of designs baseline-treatment comparisons serve as a basis for evaluating experimental findings. The accuracy of predicted changes across phases places an equally important role in evaluating the effectiveness of treatment in studies using either group of procedures. The sole but important difference between the two occurs during the second A portion of an A-B-A or A-B-A-B study. When a reversal design is employed, behavior is returned toward baseline by applying the experimental contingencies to an alternate behavior incompatible with the target behavior trained in B. Often, for example, a subject may be trained to emit a response that had been produced at a high level before intervention. Similarly, a reversal may be implemented by applying the contingencies to all non-target behaviors that occur. This schedule is sometimes referred to as differential reinforcement of other behavior (DRO).

A brief reconsideration of the Daniel and Guitar (1978) study discussed in Chapter 1 may highlight the differences between withdrawal and reversal designs. Recall that the purpose of this study was to examine the effectiveness of EMG feedback on the oral muscular activity of a subject who had undergone surgical anastomosis of the facial and hypoglossal nerves. EMG feedback was provided to the subject as an audible tone increasing in frequency as the muscular contraction increased at selected oral sites. The feedback allowed the subject to monitor his increased muscular activity by listening to the frequency of the tone. Although the authors attributed increases in oral muscular activity to EMG feedback, it was noted that this conclusion may not have been warranted because an A-B design was used rather than a single-case experimental design. It was suggested, therefore, that the authors could have strengthened their study by expanding it into an A-B-A design. A careful assessment of this suggestion, however, would have revealed that it would not have been feasible to use an A-B-A withdrawal design. Had a withdrawal been attempted, the final A phase of the study would have involved the removal of tonal feedback to determine if a decrease in the level of oral muscular activity would have resulted. Yet, if the subject had learned to maintain a high level of muscular activity during the treatment phase, removal of feedback might not alter this improvement. Therefore, an A-B-A reversal design would have been a more appropriate design. The major difference between selection of a withdrawal or reversal would have occurred during the second A phase of the A-B-A design. Instead of simply withdrawing treatment, a reversal could have been implemented by providing feedback contingent on decreases in muscle action potentials during this final phase. The same procedures and instructions used during training could have again been employed during the reversal phase. However, increases in the frequency of the tone would have been provided when the amount of muscular contraction was reduced, instead of when it was increased. If the tonal feedback had been responsible for the increase in muscular activity during the treatment (B) phase, then making feedback contingent on reduction in muscular contraction during the second A phase should result in a reversal of the treatment effect. In this way, the reversal of the experimental contingencies would have permitted an assessment of the effectiveness of the EMG feedback.

THE A-B-A-B REVERSAL DESIGN

In practice, it is not always easy to predict which target behaviors will be extinguished when a withdrawal procedure is implemented. This is particularly true in areas of research in which there are few previous examples of withdrawal designs in literature and treatment variables of interest have not been extensively studied. The following example demonstrates the practical difficulties that may be encountered in selecting an appropriate experimental design. More importantly, it highlights the flexibility of single-case experimental designs and demonstrates the practical utility of the reversal strategy.

Roll (1973) used an A-B-A-B design to examine the effect of differential visual feedback on the amount of hypernasality produced by two cleft palate subjects. The subject of interest to this discussion was a 10-year-old male with unilateral cleft of the lip, hard palate, and soft palate. After surgical repair of the cleft, a mild degree of hypernasality remained.

Hypernasality was operationally defined as "vibration of the walls of the nasal cavities during production of an English vowel or diphthong" (Roll, 1973, p. 399) and was instrumentally measured. That is, an electro-mechanical transducer was placed on the subject's nostril and nasal vibrations operated a digital counter which automatically tallied the number of nasal responses produced during each experimental phase. The production of nasal and non-nasal responses also activated electronic relays that controlled the presentation of visual feedback during treatment phases.

Experimental sessions were held five times per week in a sound-treated booth. During the baseline or "no feedback (No FB)" condition the subject was asked to "Say /eɪ/ until I ask you to stop." A total of 250 responses were produced and the nasal and non-nasal productions were accumulated on the digital counter. No instructions or feedback were provided during the baseline condition. The vowel production task and measurement techniques employed in baseline were maintained during the treatment phase, but differential visual feedback was also provided for nasal and non-nasal vowel productions. Specifically, each nasal response activated a red light mounted in front of the subject, and non-nasal vowels illuminated a white light. Instructions were also provided that asked the subject to "try to make the white light come on every time you say your sound" (p. 400). The treatment condition continued until 200 consecutive non-nasal responses had been produced. After the subject met the training criterion, a withdrawal phase (A) was introduced. Visual feedback was withdrawn and the subject was instructed to "make the response that turned the white light on without the help of the light" (p. 400). Although it was anticipated that removal of feedback would result in an increase in percentage of nasal responses, this did not occur, as the subject maintained his low rate of nasalized responding. Because the withdrawal was not successful, the authors decided to change to a reversal procedure to demonstrate experimental control, and a "feedback reversal" condition was implemented. In this condition the type of visual feedback provided was reversed from that given during the initial treatment phase, so that production of non-nasal sounds activated the red light and the white light was activated by nasal responses. As can be seen from the data that follow, the reversal of differential visual feedback was successful. Therefore, after a brief re-introduction of the "no-feedback" condition, the original treatment conditions (B) were again reinstated.

The results of this study are presented in Figure 5. It is apparent that a stable rate of responding was produced during the baseline (No FB) phase, as

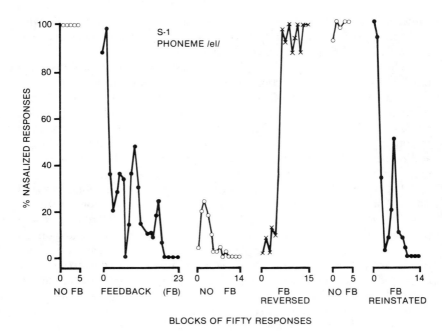

Figure 5. Percentage of /eɪ/ sounds nasalized by subject 1 on each block of 50 trials under feed-back, no-feedback, and reversed-feedback conditions. Feedback consisted of a white light produced by nonnasal responses and red light by nasal responses. (From Roll, 1973, p. 401. Copyright by Society for the Experimental Analysis of Behavior, Inc. Reproduced with permission).

100% of the vowels produced during this phase were nasalized. During the treatment condition ("feedback") there was a marked reduction in the percentage of nasalized vowel productions and no nasalized sounds were produced by the end of the treatment phase. Withdrawal is the third phase in the figure and is labeled "No Feedback." Although there was an initial increase in the percentage of nasal sounds produced during this phase, removal of treatment did not result in a reliable change in behavior. Had the study been terminated after the withdrawal phase, experimental control would not have been demonstrated and the results of the study would have been uninterpretable. Examination of the subject's performance during the "feedback reversal" phase, however, reveals that reversing the differential visual feedback resulted in a marked increase (100%) in percentage of nasalized vowels. Thus, it would appear that feedback was the primary factor in controlling the subject's nasal resonance. Inspection of the final phase supports this conclusion because reinstatement of differential visual feedback again resulted in a marked decrease in percentage of nasalized vowel responses.

It should be apparent from this example that within-subject experimental designs are both powerful and extremely flexible. Unlike group designs, single-case methodologies can be modified during the course of a study to compensate for practical problems that may arise. A conscientious investigator will, of course, attempt to control as many extraneous variables as possible and anticipate potential problems before carrying out a treatment study. However, it is not always possible to predict the difficulties that may be encountered. Single-subject research strategies put a researcher in the enviable position of being able to recognize and sometimes control problems when they occur.

In the preceding sections withdrawal and reversal designs were used to demonstrate control over behaviors being emitted at a high rate of production. Quite often, however, it is desirable to shape a behavior not in a subject's repertoire, or to increase the rate of a behavior only minimally present. For example, an investigator may wish to shape a distorted articulatory response into an acoustically acceptable one or train a language-impaired subject to use appropriate tense markers. In any event, the applicability of A-B-A-B designs is not restricted to demonstrating control over behaviors being produced more frequently than is desirable for efficient communication. The following example demonstrates this point and further emphasizes the methodology of the A-B-A-B reversal design.

Jackson and Wallace (1974) attempted to increase the vocal intensity level of a 15-year-old mentally retarded girl who "almost never spoke at an audible level." The investigation was initiated after previous attempts to modify her loudness level had been unsuccessful. Throughout the investigation the subject was seated in a plywood cubicle lined with acoustical tile.

A portable neck-level microphone activated a voice-operated relay and controlled delivery of tokens during the appropriate experimental phases. The experimenter manually controlled the sensitivity of the voice-operated relay and monitored the intensity of the subject's responses on the sound level meter. All of the subject's responses were tape recorded.

During the baseline phase, the subject was presented with 100 stimulus cards with single monosyllabic words written on them. She was instructed to read the cards while the experimenter recorded the intensity of each response on the sound level meter. No feedback or consequences were presented during the six baseline sessions. After baseline, a treatment phase was initiated in which tokens were presented contingent upon reading responses of sufficient intensity to operate the voice-activated relay. Specific instructions requested that the subject "talk loudly and earn a lot of tokens" (p. 463).

Throughout this phase the experimenter decreased the sensitivity of the voice-operated relay whenever "approximately 80% of the subject's responses operated the relay and token delivery mechanism" (p. 463). Each adjustment required the subject to produce louder responses in order to obtain tokens.

The reversal phase of this study was implemented after termination of the treatment phase. During this condition the token contingencies were reversed so that decreases in loudness were consequated. That is, tokens were delivered each time a stimulus word was read softly enough to avoid activating the voice-operated relay. The subject was "gradually required to speak softer and softer...even though the instructions given by the experimenter continued to indicate otherwise" (p. 463). The final phase of the study consisted of reinstatement of the initial treatment condition in which the subject was consequated for increases in vocal intensity. Although a follow-up training condition was also implemented, it is not relevant to the current discussion and will not be considered.

The results of this study are presented in Figure 6. It can be seen that the data are presented relative to the average loudness levels produced by five peer subjects. The comparison group had received the "exact conditions" that prevailed for the subject during the baseline phase. Before treatment (A), the subject's average intensity level was consistently below the mean level produced by the peer comparison group (0). Initiation of the "tokens for louder speech" phase (B) resulted in a gradual increase in the loudness level until it equalled the peer group's average by the fortieth treatment session. This trend toward increased loudness continued throughout the treatment condition, eventually even surpassing the subjects in the highest range of the peer group. The loudness level of the experimental subject's reading responses fell dramatically during the reversal condition (A). Presentation of "tokens for softer speech" reduced her intensity to a level that approximated the average of the comparison group. Finally, reinstatement of the "tokens for louder speech" phase (B), again resulted in an obvious increase in loudness level. These results were taken to support "the hypothesis that the token contingency had been a significant variable in increasing the subject's voice loudness" (p. 465).

As in the discussions of the previous studies, a brief consideration of methodological aspects of this study may be enlightening. The authors carefully described their instrumentation, the experimental setting, and general methodology. For example, each experimental session consisted of 100 single-word reading responses and each response within a session was cued by the onset of a signal light. However, several specific procedural ambiguities detract from the overall replicability of the study. Specifically,

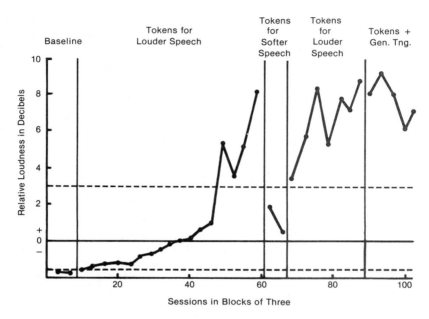

Figure 6. Results of the "shaping" sessions, in blocks of three sessions per data point. The data are shown in relation to the average loudness of the subject's peers in this setting (zero point on the ordinate). The range for these subjects is shown by the dashed line. After baseline, tokens were given for meeting a loudness or softness criterion. Additional procedures were used in the final experimental phase to ensure behavior change in the classroom. (From Jackson and Wallace, 1974, p. 465. Copyright by Society for the Experimental Analysis of Behavior, Inc. Reproduced with permission.)

criterion for changing response levels (approximately 80%) was loosely specified and there were no criteria reported for termination of any of the experimental phases. Establishing criteria for baseline, training, and reversal phases would have clarified and objectified the experimental procedure. Similarly, it should be noted that no inter-judge reliability was obtained during the A-B-A-B phases on the experimenter's ability to record the loudness data from the decibel meter. Although adequate reliability data were reported for contextual reading generalization probes, this does not ensure that the experimenter accurately recorded the intensity data during the experimental sessions. The unique method of presenting the data in this study is also of interest. Due to the length of the study, the data were averaged across blocks of three sessions. Although this was a necessity in this study, averaging should be avoided whenever possible so that any variability or trends in the data are easily discernible. Another unique aspect of the data presentation in this study is that the results are graphed relative to the performance of a peer group. This is unusual in that actual, rather than relative, data are generally presented for within-subject studies because the process of graphically showing changes in the actual behavior treated facilitates interpretation of results and avoids unnecessary inferences about performance. In exercising their prerogative to present their data relative to a comparison group, Jackson and Wallace (1974) seem to have added some valuable information. The peer group does not truly provide "a norm of voice loudness" as the authors suggest it does, yet, it provides additional perspective with regard to the clinical significance of the data. (See Social Validation, chapter 4). However, it should again be emphasized that there was not replication of this study across subjects. Therefore, one cannot assess the generality of the results. A number of the issues raised by this study, including the need to establish adequate performance criteria, reliability data presentation, and replication are further discussed in chapters 4 and 5 of this text.

Reversal and withdrawal designs share the same limitations. Both tend to be more time consuming and, therefore, more costly than other within-subject experimental designs. In addition, resistance may be encountered when cooperation is enlisted from professionals who are not familiar with the logic or power of these designs. Reversal designs do, however, offer several noteworthy advantages over withdrawal designs. Reversals are less time consuming than their withdrawal counterparts, because implementation of reversal training procedures may avoid lengthy periods of extinction that sometimes occur when withdrawal designs are employed. In addition, reversal designs are advantageous when the target behaviors are likely to be resistive to extinction. One final advantage of reversal designs relates to the availability of consequation during the reversal phase (Sulzer-Azaroff and Mayer, 1977). Whereas all contingencies are removed when a withdrawal design is utilized, contingencies may be applied to nontarget behaviors when a reversal is implemented. As a result, the availability of consequation may help to maintain a high level of subject participation throughout a reversal phase.

SUMMARY AND CONCLUDING REMARKS

After consideration of several basic principles that underlie within-subject designs, the withdrawal and reversal designs have been distinguished and examples presented to demonstrate the A-B-A, B-A-B and A-B-A-B designs. Advantages and limitations of each design strategy have been presented.

During our discussion of reversal designs it was noted that they have several additional benefits that are not inherent in withdrawal designs and one might infer that reversals have wider applicability to the area of communicative disorders than withdrawal designs. Unlike withdrawal designs they provide a means of overcoming the effects of environmental influences when they are present. Given the innumerable settings in which trained communicative behaviors may be inadvertently modeled and consequated, a forced reversal is likely to be an important experimental manipulation in this area of research. It should be kept in mind, however, that the implementation of a reversal may be procedurally more complex than a withdrawal because of the additional training involved, and the appropriateness of an experimental design will ultimately be determined by the behavior being studied and the specific question posed.

Despite the power and elegance of withdrawal and reversal designs, some investigators may be reluctant to employ these research strategies. Leitenberg (1973), for example, notes an apparently common fear that once training is withdrawn or reversed behavior may be difficult to retrain. This fear does not appear to be justified, however, because studies from a variety of applied behavioral disciplines indicate that if a treatment is powerful enough to train a behavior initially, it will be powerful enough to retrain that same behavior. A more legitimate concern for the researcher deciding on a single-case design relates to problems encountered when withdrawal and reversal procedures are implemented.

Reversal and withdrawal designs provide a powerful means of demonstrating experimental control over an individual behavior and they have occasionally been used to examine the effects of treatment variables on small groups of subjects, such as all students in a given classroom. However, like all designs, they are not appropriate for some types of experimental situations. Specifically, some behaviors, such as auditory discrimination, may not be reversible and alternative strategies would be needed to explore questions about this topic. In addition, practical or ethical considerations prevent the use of a withdrawal or reversal design. One practical limitation, the fact that these designs are more time consuming than other within-subject designs, has been discussed previously. Ethical considerations that preclude using these designs are, however, also noteworthy. It may, for example, be undesirable or ethically objectionable to reverse a subject's performance to his baseline level if the behavior under study is detrimental to him or her or to others in a personally or socially significant manner. Thus, after training a particular functional communication skill, which helps a mentally retarded individual better integrate into a noninstitutional environment, one might not want to extinguish the trained behavior. Similarly, if a training program has been used to reduce the excessive amount of swearing (coprolalia) exhibited by a subject with Gilles de la Tourette syndrome, an investigator would probably be reluctant to increase the use of antisocial language by using a reversal procedure.

Finally, one additional limitation of withdrawal and reversal designs deserves mention. These types of design strategies should be avoided whenever treatment effects are expected to carry over across experimental phases.

When the above factors rule out the use of withdrawal or reversal strategies, multiple-baseline designs provide an attractive option. The use of multiple-baseline design is discussed in Chapter 3.

Multiple-
Baseline
Designs

3

A common substitute for the A-B-A or A-B-A-B is a multiple-baseline design. It is especially useful when the behavior is irreversible or should not be reversed for ethical reasons. An example of an irreversible behavior would be responses to a speech sound discrimination task. Once a subject has learned to discriminate between two sounds, the behavior cannot be reversed. An example of a behavior that, ethically, should not be reversed would be self-punishment acts by an autistic child. If a treatment has been effective in extinguishing the self-punishment or replacing it with a more socially acceptable behavior, the experimenter would be loath to reverse contingencies to increase self-punishment again. A multiple-baseline design circumvents these problems by omitting the reversal phase of the design entirely.

The basic components of a multiple-baseline design are explained in this chapter. For illustrative purposes, a multiple-baseline across behaviors is used. However, several forms of the design are available, for example, multiple-baseline across subjects or settings. These alternative forms are described later in the chapter. Examples from the communicative disorders literature are presented to illustrate how the designs have been used to investigate treatment of communicative disorders.

MULTIPLE-BASELINE ACROSS BEHAVIORS

As in other single-subject experimental designs, the A and B components are basic to the multiple-baseline design. The A component must meet the same criteria in a multiple-baseline design that it does in an A-B-A design. That is, the behavior to be treated must be defined operationally and measured at length to demonstrate stability before treatment. When stability criteria have been met, treatment is initiated and administered in B until the behavior change meets the criteria set by the experimenter. In a multiple baseline design, however, a second A phase is not required to extinguish or to reverse the behavior obtained in the B phase.

Control in a multiple-baseline design comes from a replication of treatment effects on another behavior (or subject, etc.), not a reversal or withdrawal of treatment on the first behavior, although that may occur also. Hence, the label *multiple-baseline across behaviors,* means that more than one behavior is treated in the design. The same treatment is applied to all selected behaviors but treatments are administered to the behaviors in sequence. A multiple-baseline design involving two behaviors is illustrated in Figure 7.

In a multiple-baseline across two behaviors, the purpose is to determine if a single treatment is effective in changing two behaviors in the same way in one subject. The two behaviors selected for treatment need to be different enough from one another that treatment of one does not influence the other until it receives treatment. On the other hand, the two behaviors cannot be so different that a single treatment is inapplicable to both.

Initially, a baseline measurement is taken on both behaviors. When stability criterion is reached on the two behaviors, treatment is started on the

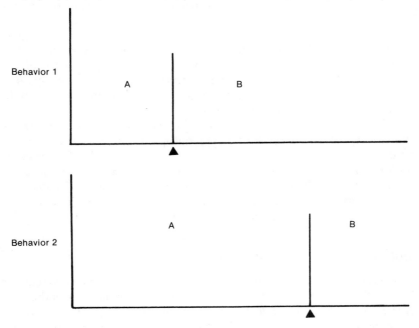

Figure 7. The design for a multiple-baseline study involving two behaviors.

first one. The second behavior continues in baseline while the first is treated. When treatment on the first behavior is completed, treatment is shifted to the second behavior until a behavioral change has been demonstrated. It is assumed that the second behavior will continue to show stability in the protracted baseline measurement until treatment for the first behavior is terminated. It is the second behavior that imparts the experimental control in a multiple-baseline that is achieved by a reversal in the A-B-A design. If the second behavior does not change while the first is in treatment, this stability demonstrates that the independent variable (treatment) affects only the dependent variable (behavior) to which it is applied. The stable baseline in the second behavior also demonstrates that time, maturation, and other extraneous variables are not changing the behavior before application of the independent variable. If these events were operating on the first behavior and confounding the results, they would also be operating on the second behavior, with the result that the second behavior would change before treatment is administered, during the extensive baseline. Consequently, if the second behavior remains unaltered throughout the period in which the first behavior is treated, then confounding variables are not operating during treatment, or if they are operating, they are not influencing the behavior treated. To assure that this is so, application of the independent variable to the second behavior, after the first behavior has been treated, must result in a change in the second behavior. This is an essential component to demonstrate control. The second behavior must change in a way similar to the first behavior in treatment. If it does not, then the effect of the independent variable has not been shown and the study reverts to a simple A-B design without the necessary experimental controls. In a successful multiple-baseline design there are two points of evidence for experimental control. These points are indicated by arrows in Figure 7. The first point occurs at the conjunction between the end of the baseline and the beginning of treatment of the first behavior. The second point occurs at the baseline-treatment conjunction of the second behavior. In both cases, behavior changed only when treatment was administered. In this way, the second behavior serves a replication purpose for demonstrating treatment effectiveness.

To illustrate application of a multiple-baseline design across two behaviors, a hypothetical study is described. The description does not include details of the study procedures to prevent obscuring the purpose of the illustration. It is assumed that appropriate definitions, measurements, instrumentation, and procedures are present; emphasis is placed on design components.

Assume that an experimenter has designed, or has obtained, an instrument on which the acoustic features composing the sounds of English are displayed visually. Each sound has a characteristic outline or form as a result of its features, and a standard form for each sound is available by pressing the appropriate button. The visual form can be maintained on the screen until a button press removes it. If the sound is produced into a microphone while the form is maintained on the screen, the characteristics of the production are superimposed on the form already present on the screen, allowing an examination of the two forms to determine how well they match.

The experimenter wishes to explore whether this instrument can be used in helping children with cleft palates produce accurate plosive and fricative sounds, sounds frequently in error in cleft-palate children. Furthermore, if the treatment proves effective, the experimenter will wish to know if the accurate responses continue after treatment is terminated.

The visual display is to be used in the form of feedback. The experimenter pushes the button for a specific sound so that the standard form is displayed on the screen. The child is requested to produce the same sound, trying to match the form on the screen. The feedback for the sound production is closeness of the match between the standard and the form produced by the subject. The instrument is equipped to print out pluses and minuses for matches and nonmatches. The pluses and minuses compose the data for determining the number of correct responses produced by the child. The dependent variable is correct sound production as defined by a match of the standard and the child's form read out as pluses and minuses on paper tape. The independent variable is the feedback received by viewing superimposition of the child's own form on the standard and checking the closeness of the match.

To investigate the effectiveness of the feedback the experimenter uses a multiple-baseline design. Two sounds are selected to represent two classes of sounds, the /p/ represents plosives and the /s/ represents fricatives. The design for the study is shown in Figure 8.

The two behaviors studied are the two sounds, /p/ and /s/. The single treatment to be applied to both is feedback in the form of a visual match.

In baseline procedures the subject sits in front of the screen. Displayed on the screen is the visual form of either the standard for /p/ or /s/. The experimenter turns the form on for 15 seconds and asks the child to produce the sound. After 15 seconds the standard is turned off and the screen is blank for 5 seconds before the standard is presented again. The child's production is not displayed on the screen, but the match or mismatch of the two productions is recorded by the instrument. Each baseline session consists of 60 trials. On half of the trials the /p/ is presented and the /s/ is presented on the remaining trials. Baseline for the two sounds extends over four sessions and presentation of the two sounds is alternated over sessions.

When baseline shows that no correct responses were recorded for either sound, the experimenter initiates training on /p/ in the fifth session. Now

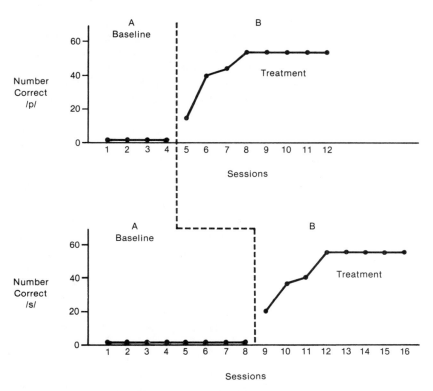

Figure 8. A multiple-baseline design for investigating the effect of feedback on /p/ and /s/ production.

the subject views the matches and mismatches each time he produces /p/. After 60 training trials on /p/ are completed in a session, the feedback is turned off, the /s/ standard presented, and the child is requested to produce the /s/ a total of 60 times without feedback as in the first four baseline sessions.

Training on /p/ is continued for four sessions. In each session the child receives 60 training trials on /p/ and 60 baseline trials on /s/. After the eighth session has been completed (assuming no major problems have arisen) treatment is shifted to /s/. The protracted baseline on /s/ has continued to show no correct /s/ productions, so it is possible to apply the treatment to the second baseline behavior. Now, each time the child produces /s/, the form is superimposed on the standard /s/ form on the screen and he observes the closeness of the match. Training for /s/ is identical to the /p/ training and is continued for four sessions just as in /p/ training.

The above is a somewhat simplistic, but nevertheless basic description of a multiple-baseline design. The design is fundamental in the presence of the major components, and as previously explained, control is demonstrated in the changes in behavior that occur for each behavior as a shift in conditions from baseline to treatment is made; changes occur only when treatment is initiated. The above description concerns the major components and variations within the basic format are possible.

For example, one might reasonably inquire what occurs in the four sessions after treatment is terminated. In Figure 8 the /p/ phase continues for 12 sessions, although treatment terminates at 8, and in the /s/ phase, 16 sessions are planned, although treatment ended in session 12. Several possibilities are available to the experimenter in designing a multiple-baseline study. A design will conform to the questions posed by the investigator. Unlike the hypothetical study, an experimenter may choose to end the study when training is completed if the purpose of the study is merely to examine the direct effect of the independent variable as it is applied over a specified period of time.

At times, however, experimenters will wish to explore further. For instance, they may wish to continue the treatment on the first behavior even when shifting to the second behavior to study if effectiveness continues over a longer period of time. This can be readily arranged while treatment is applied to the second behavior. Thus, after treatment is initiated on /s/, the experimenter may continue treatment on /p/ so that both sounds are receiving feedback simultaneously. The experimenter must be cautious in deciding whether treatment on the first behavior should continue if he entertains any possibility of confounding treatment of the second behavior by this continuation. If confounding is suspected, it is safer to discontinue treatment on the first behavior when the independent variable is applied to the second behavior. In the hypothetical study, the experimenter would weigh the risks carefully. If continuing to provide feedback on /p/ productions during /s/ training presents a problem in interfering with /s/ training, the /p/ feedback should be terminated after the eighth session. Measurement of /p/ productions can also be discontinued because the /p/ phase of the experiment is concluded when training is shifted to /s/.

Other times the experimenter wishes to study maintenance effects of a treatment after treatment has been terminated. Such was the desire of the experimenter in the hypothetical study, as will be recalled. Not only was the experiment designed to explore the effect of the feedback on accuracy of /p/ and /s/ production, but more, it was designed to explore whether treatment effects were maintained past the period in which treatment was administered. To this end, four additional measurement sessions were designed for each sound.

These four sessions resemble the second A phase in an A-B-A study in which treatment is withdrawn to demonstrate that the response trained in B will extinguish when treatment is removed. In an A-B-A study, the withdrawal phase is the control phase—and it is essential that the response be extinguished or experimental control is lost and results remain inconclusive. Usually, the experimenter has some prior indications from experience, previous studies, and so on, that if the treatment is withdrawn the response will probably be extinguished, and, therefore, a reversal design might be suitable.

Just the opposite possibility is inherent in choosing a multiple-baseline design. In this case the experimenter, taking into account all factors, concludes that there is a strong likelihood that the response will be maintained after treatment is withdrawn; therefore, an A-B-A design is unsuitable, and a multiple-baseline design offers a better possibility for demonstrating treatment effects. Partly to test these intuitions and partly to measure the degree of maintenance, the experimenter designs the study to extend beyond the termination of treatment. In the hypothetical feedback study the experimenter's knowledge leads him to suspect that the correct production, if acquired during training, would be retained after feedback stopped. It was desirable to measure the extent of the maintenance; consequently, four additional sessions similar to baseline procedures for both sounds were included in the study design.

It is not always feasible to study maintenance in the absence of any training, for a variety of reasons. Primarily, the behavior may indeed be lost and this would be an undesirable development, or the experimenter would prefer to maintain the behavior at a high level, so an event is programmed into the maintenance phase to increase the probability that the behavior is maintained. The event may take a form not used during training, or it could be the same event used in training, but be presented less often during maintenance sessions. Returning to the feedback study, the experimenter could shift from the visual display as feedback to verbal praise for correct responses offered intermittently by the experimenter. This would be an example of a new event.

It is more likely that the experimenter would be more comfortable in retaining the same treatment, but presenting it intermittently rather than continuously. Possibly, after training shifted to /s/, the experimenter could present visual feedback to the subject on /p/ only on every tenth trial with the hope that six trials of feedback per session are sufficient to maintain a high level of accurate production for four sessions. No experimental question is posed regarding the maintenance phase, controls to study the effect of six feedback trials were not planned into the design; the experimenter merely wishes to collect data in this phase. If the data warrant further exploration, a proper study could be designed.

Length of Phases

Notice that in the feedback study the length of the phases was kept constant and equal; four sessions of baseline, four sessions of treatment, and four sessions of maintenance. Furthermore, the number of trials within sessions was identical across all sessions. That is the advantage of using hypothetical examples; they can be made to depict the ideal design.

Reasons for the equality are self-evident. If treatment continues for a longer period than baseline it is possible to wonder if variables are operating in treatment that were not operating in baseline. It is Hersen and Barlow's (1976) suggestion that the phases be kept equal. Unfortunately, the equality criterion poses practical problems for experimenters investigating communicative disorders, as noted in Chapter 2.

Therefore, most experimenters prefer to set a criterion level as a cutoff point in treatment rather than specify the number of sessions to be devoted to treatment before terminating the condition. This, of course, is because of the problems encountered in making accurate guesses about the course of treatment in communicative disorders. For example, it is not possible to state with any certainty that a child with a cleft palate will learn to produce /p/ or /s/ in four sessions (although our hypothetical experimenter appears confident enough). It is a reasonable guess, but acquisition of articulation is usually a gradual progression through a series of approximations that remain unidentified and therefore unpredictable, except in broad terms. The range of possibilities makes experimenters in communicative disorders reluctant to set limits to training except within reasonable bounds. The preference is to set criterion levels and train until criterion is reached or until a reasonable number of trials have been administered before terminating treatment. Setting criterion levels for shifting conditions almost always results in an unequal number of sessions in the various phases of the experiment. The experimenter decides which is most important to the study, keeping all phases of the experiment equal, or giving the treatment ample opportunity to have an effect on the behavior, even if it means unequal phases. When an experimenter feels confident in his or her prediction of time or trials it should take to demonstrate effectiveness, the design, assuredly, should be planned with an equal number of sessions in each condition.

A second advantage of using equal phases is the comparative ease with which comparisons between conditions can be made. Session-by-session comparison provides a clear picture of the course of treatment in comparison to the sessions spent in measuring baseline.

Counterbalancing

Whenever more than one behavior is treated sequentially, there is risk of order effects. In the feedback study, training on /s/ followed training on /p/. Undoubtedly, the two behaviors were different enough to require independent treatment, but *order effects* refers to more than similarity in the behaviors trained. It is plausible that /s/ production was learned with the feedback primarily because /p/ had first been learned with the feedback. Conceivably, had /s/ been trained first, the child may not have learned it. This conjecture appears unreasonable on the surface; nevertheless, the possibility cannot be discounted. Order effects are touched on in Chapter 1 in the discussion of one treatment following another in an A-B or B study. It is not possible to know if the third treatment in the Brookner and Murphy (1975) study was successful just because the child had received prior training (Chapter 1). In the same way, in a multiple-baseline study, perhaps the first feedback training was teaching the child to learn to use feedback, a prerequisite to producing an accurate /s/ when it was trained later. Such order effects can be ruled out in multiple-baseline studies and this is accomplished through counterbalancing.

Counterbalancing requires a second subject who serves to counter order effects by going through the experiment in an opposite order from the first subject, thus balancing the order of the behaviors trained. The feedback study requires an additional subject to counterbalance the order effects of /p/ training first and /s/ training second. The second subject would receive reverse training; training on /s/ first and on /p/ second. In that way, any order effects are controlled. The complete multiple-baseline design would show the counterbalancing, as in Figure 9.

Whereas in A-B-A designs replications are desirable, particularly if generality is sought, in multiple-baseline designs they are mandatory, although all researchers would not emphasize this aspect of the design (Hersen and Barlow, 1976). On the subject of replications, a direct replication of any study conducted on a single subject is now common. Seldom are studies involving only one subject considered sufficient. The demand is for a replication of the effect on at least one other subject. Thus, the term single-subject studies, if taken literally, is a misnomer.

Selecting Behaviors

Previously it was mentioned that the two behaviors selected for treatment in a multiple-baseline study must be different enough that they can be treated in-

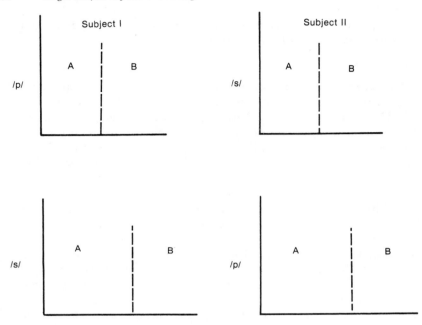

Figure 9. A multiple-baseline design with counterbalancing for order effects in exploring the effect of feedback on /p/ and /s/ production.

dependently, and yet similar enough that the treatment can be applied to both. In communicative disorders this means that the investigator must select judiciously because the interrelationships in verbal and vocal behaviors are frequently strong ones.

Let us take an example by returning to the hypothetical study of the /p/ and /s/ sound training. The two sounds were selected because they are highly dissimilar in that they share very few features. The /p/ is a plosive, discontinuant, nonstrident, and unvoiced sound. The /s/ is a fricative, continuant, strident, and unvoiced sound. The only feature the two sounds share is unvoicing. The selection was based partly on the dissimilarity in features, and partly on the basis of studies showing that generalization does not occur between the two sounds. That is, if one is trained, the other does not change. They are sufficiently distant from each other not to affect one another. Yet, they are both speech sounds; and feedback, albeit a different kind of feedback, should be necessary to learn to produce both. The different kind of feedback refers not to the procedure used, but to the acoustic characteristics composing each sound, the forms illuminated on the screen.

The investigator would probably have encountered a problem had he selected /s/ and /z/ as the two sounds for training. These two sounds share all features, except voicing. Additionally, generalization studies show that training on /s/ results in changes on /z/. Undoubtedly, training on /s/ would have resulted in a loss of the /z/ baseline in the training study in that as /s/ training progressed, /z/ production would have gradually improved. The two sounds are too similar for a multiple-baseline design, which requires independent treatment of each behavior.

A problem would also have been encountered if the investigator had selected to train two different parameters of vocal behavior, say, rate of /s/ production and acoustic (visual) characteristics of /p/. The problem is obvious; the instrument is not equipped to provide rate feedback. Such feedback would require different treatment. The principle of two different behaviors and a single treatment would have been destroyed in that situation.

It is not always easy to know which behaviors are amenable to investigation in a multiple-baseline design. As mentioned, selection may require careful judgment. The experimenter relies on published descriptive data, and on studies in which the two behaviors have been trained and generalization between them tested. Finally, he or she relies on experiences in the clinic or laboratory in which the two behaviors have been observed.

Multiple-Baseline Across Two Behaviors

Bennett's study (1974) of two hearing-impaired children was designed as a multiple-baseline experiment across behaviors. The children misarticulated fricatives, and the two selected for study were the /f/ and /ʃ/. The investigator's purpose was to determine if the procedures would be effective in training the children to produce the sounds correctly, and if the corrected sounds would generalize to untrained words containing them. Nine words were selected for each sound, one for training and eight for probing. The training word contained the /f/ or /ʃ/ in initial position (e.g., fox and shop), five of the probe words contained the sounds in the initial position of words (e.g., fire and ship), and three in the final position of words (e.g., leaf and dish).

The two 4-year-old girls were profoundly and severely hearing impaired. The multiple baseline consisted of the words containing the two sounds, that is, the /f/ and /ʃ/ words. Baseline 1 included /f/ words, and baseline 2 included the /ʃ/ words. Pictures accompanied the words (e.g., picture of ship for the word ship). For both girls, the first sound trained was the /f/ in the word fox. After /f/, training was shifted to /ʃ/ in the word shop. Thus, the sequential training of the two sounds formed the multiple-baseline design.

Prior to any training a baseline was obtained on both sounds. Baseline consisted of presentation of the eight /f/ pictures and eight /ʃ/ pictures used in the probes for spontaneous naming by children. The training words (fox and shop) were not presented during baseline measurement. The five pictures with the sound in the initial position were presented twice, whereas the three pictures with the sound in the final position were presented three times in each baseline session. These baseline sessions were administered on consecutive days.

Training procedures were divided into two phases, an imitation and spontaneous production phase. In imitation, the appropriate picture was presented, the experimenter named the picture, and the child was required to imitate the model presented by the experimenter. When criterion was reached in the imitation phase, the spontaneous phase was initiated. In this phase the experimenter held up the picture and asked the child to name it. All correct responses in both phases were followed by tokens (later exchanged for candy) and a verbal "good." When criterion in the spontaneous phase was reached, a probe of the remaining untrained words was administered. The probe included the eight untrained words containing /f/, the training sound, as well as the eight words containing /ʃ/, the sound not yet trained. The procedures in probing were the same as those used in baseline testing with no consequent event for correct or incorrect productions. If at least seven of the words containing the training sound were produced correctly, generalization criterion was considered to have been met. After the probe, training was shifted to the /ʃ/ training word. When training criterion was met on <u>shop</u>, the /f/ and /ʃ/ untrained words were presented again to check for generalization.

Results for the two children are presented in Figures 10 and 11. The results are presented somewhat differently from the way multiple-baseline design results are commonly presented (refer to Figure 7 on page 52 for usual portrayal of multiple-baseline design results). As the data show, when the children were trained on /f/ in <u>fox</u>, they achieved criterion in both training phases. The probe at the end of /f/ spontaneous training showed that both children had generalized to the /f/ initial position words at a high level, less so to the final /f/ words; there was no change from baseline in the /ʃ/ words for either child. After the first probe, training on /ʃ/ was initiated in the word <u>shop</u>. When criterion in spontaneous training was reached all the untrained words were presented again. On this final probe Sue generalized to the /ʃ/ words and maintained correct responding on the /f/ words. Mich correctly produced the /ʃ/ and /f/ in initial position words in the second probe, but evidenced no change on the words with the /f/ and /ʃ/ in the final position. The experimenter concluded that "operant procedures can be effectively used to teach hearing-impaired children to articulate correctly the phonemes /f/ and /ʃ/ in the initial position of words. The training procedures. . .facilitated generalization of the target phonemes to other words requiring these phonemes in the initial position and final position of words on which the girls had received no training" (p. 444).

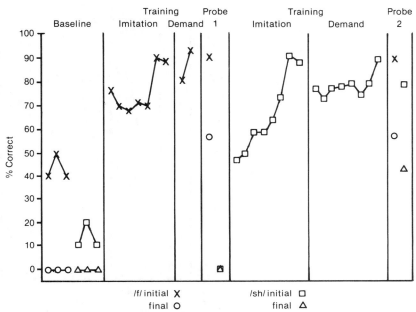

Figure 10. Percentage of responses correct at baseline for the imitation and demand training sets and two probes for Sue. Each data point during training represents 50 trials. (From Bennett, 1974, p. 442. Copyright by the Society for the Experimental Analysis of Behavior, Inc. Reproduced with permission).

Results of the study attest to the successful execution of the multiple-baseline design. The second behavior (/ʃ/ production) did not change until treatment was applied to it. Several aspects of the study deserve comment, however, because in some ways the design is atypical.

Recall that Bennett stated two purposes for the study. One was to determine if the subjects could be taught to articulate /f/ and /ʃ/ correctly, and the other to test generalization of the phonemes to untrained words. From the author's conclusions it appeared that the first purpose addressed the effectiveness of the training procedure and the second addressed whether the sounds changed in untrained words as a result of training. Thus, the study had two dependent variables: acquisition and generalization. Strictly speaking, data for the first question are incomplete because baseline was not taken on the /f/ in fox and /ʃ/ in shop. Although it is highly probable that the sounds were produced incorrectly in the training items before training, data to support the probability would have been helpful, enabling a controlled comparison between what was produced before and during training. It is customary to obtain baseline measures on all dependent variable responses, in this case, production of the /f/ and /ʃ/ in training and generalization

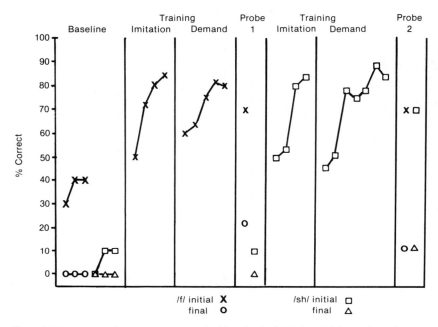

Figure 11. Percentage of responses correct at baseline for the imitation and demand training sets and two probes for Mich. Each data point during training represents 50 trials. (From Bennett, 1974, p. 443. Copyright by the Society for the Experimental Analysis of Behavior, Inc. Reproduced with permission).

items. Also, ideally, the word shop would continue to be tested during training of fox to assure that it was not changing as fox was being acquired. The high level of correct responding in the initial training session for both sounds suggests the need for baseline data on fox and shop production. Thus, the multiple-baseline was composed of the generalization items instead of a combination of the training and generalization items.

Another component in this study that differs from the components explained on pages 51 to 59 is that the second behavior (/ʃ/ words) was not measured continuously during training of the first response (fox). It is not uncommon in multiple-baseline studies of communication disorders for intermittent rather than continuous monitoring of the second baseline. In the Bennett study the second behavior was remeasured only after training for the first behavior had been completed. At times infrequent monitoring is a necessity, but if possible, the second behavior should be measured often. More frequent measurement provides more evidence for the control that is a major component of a multiple-baseline design. We hasten to point out that the lack of continuous monitoring of the second baseline does not invalidate the results of the Bennett study. Such monitoring, however, would have strengthened the design and the results.

One desirable component of a multiple-baseline design is absent in the Bennett study, and that is counterbalancing across the two behaviors. Counterbalancing could have been important because the two sounds trained were fricatives, meaning that they shared a number of articulatory characteristics. The shared features made the /ʃ/ vulnerable to influence from the previous /f/ training. Possibly, the /ʃ/ was learned partly because it was preceded by a period of training on /f/. Because both subjects were trained on /f/ first, there is no evidence that order effects were eliminated. This indicates the study was vulnerable to order effects, not that they were present. Evidence that order effects did not occur could have been presented by starting one child on /f/ training followed by /ʃ/ training and the other on /ʃ/ training followed by /f/ training. Replication of the orders would have added two more subjects, a total of four children for an ideal multiple-baseline design study of two behaviors. (More will be said about number of subjects in multiple-baseline studies). It has been mentioned before and bears repeating: counterbalancing is not considered equally crucial by all researchers, but without it, order effects cannot be ruled out.

Naturally, the components described on pages 51 and 59 are basic, but all are not equally inviolable and Bennett chose to vary some according to his needs. It is worthwhile to keep in mind which components can be changed without harming the controls built into the design, and which cannot be changed because the change would violate the design to the extent that the results would be invalid. Some changes may improve designs whereas others may impair them.

The two-behavior multiple-baseline study is possibly the most simple to design, insofar as it allows an easy examination for presence of components. All multiple-baseline studies are not equally open to evaluation without *careful* scrutiny. Modifications of the two-behavior multiple-baseline study include multiple baselines across three or more behaviors and multiple baselines across individuals and settings. Multiple baselines across subjects and groups are also possible. The variations are described in following subsections.

Three or More Behaviors

A multiple-baseline design may be sequenced across any number of behaviors. For example, returning to the hypothetical study with cleft palate children, if the instrument used for feedback were programmed to display all English sounds, the experimenter might wish to study additional sound classes, say, nasals and affricates (provided each remained independent of the others). If two more sound classes were added, the experimenter would have a four-behavior multiple-baseline study for each subject as shown in Figure 12. If counterbalancing is planned to control for order effects, however, the effect of /p/ training on /s/ would have to be considered; the effect of /p/ and /s/, and /s/ alone on /n/ training would need controlling, and so forth, through all four sound classes. All possible permutations of orders would require a total of 24 subjects. For instance, just to account for all orders when /p/ is trained first, the following six arrangements are obligatory:

$$p,s,n,t,\int$$
$$p,n,t,\int,s$$
$$p,t,\int,s,n$$
$$p,s,t,\int,n$$
$$p,t,\int,n,s$$
$$p,n,s,t,\int$$

Six similar arrangements for each of the four sounds, 24 orders, would achieve total counterbalancing; hence the need for 24 subjects. The requirement is prohibitive, of course, and investigators usually do not attempt to cover all possible orders, preferring to design a few random orders to take care of the problem. No matter how it is accomplished, however, a four-behavior multiple-baseline study requires several subjects. Needless to say, the advantages of within-subject control are diminished somewhat when too many behaviors are studied in one experiment, simply because of the number of subjects required if counterbalancing and replication are planned. With an increased subject population subject characteristics begin to pose a problem threatening to form a confounding variable. To prevent the problem, subjects can be matched as closely as possible. On the other hand, matching may become more difficult as the subject population is increased. Practically speaking, it seems less time consuming and more efficient to restrict a study to two behaviors instead of attempting to explore several at once. Replication might serve this purpose better. Yet, it is not uncommon to find three- and four-behavior multiple-baseline studies. Inasmuch as they are possibly more plentiful than two-behavior studies, it may be useful to examine one from the literature.

An interesting example of a three-behavior multiple-baseline design is found in a study by Kotkin, Simpson, and DeSanto (1978). The study was selected because it has an unusual feature. The investigators wished to explore the effect of sign language on picture naming. Two retarded children served as subjects. The multiple-baseline design consisted of three words for each subject; the words were names for pictures. The names were selected from an array of names because the children did not produce them in picture naming. For subject 1 the words were "camel," "bat," and "seal," and for subject 2 they were "watermelon," "worm," and "tomato."

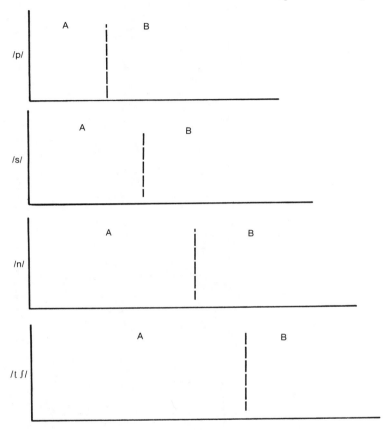

Figure 12. A multiple-baseline design across four behaviors (four speech sounds) using feedback as the treatment.

The subjects met the following selection criteria: 1) they demonstrated an understanding of the question, "What's this?," 2) they demonstrated imitation of the signs used in the experiment, and 3) they verbally imitated the words used in the experiment. The design and data for the experiment are displayed in Figure 13.

The design had the unique feature of a pre-baseline (PB) phase. Actually, this phase was used for selecting the training words, but it was also used to measure the dependent variable, which was verbally naming the pictures spontaneously to the query, "What's this?" The dependent variable was naming the three pictures spontaneously; the independent variable consisted of two training procedures, imitation of a verbal model and imitation of a sign-verbal model.

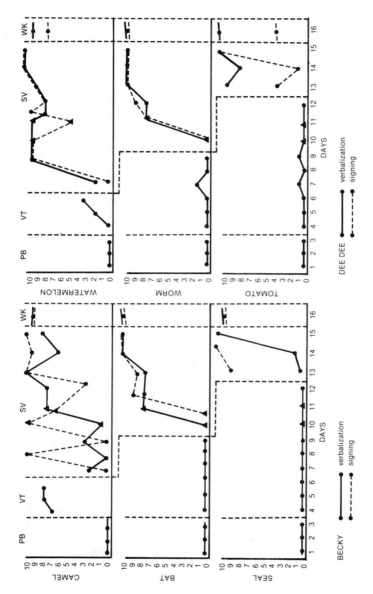

Figure 13. The number of correct verbal and signed responses during daily probes. The first segment shows the pre-baseline (PB) for selection of training words. The second segment shows verbal training only (VT). The third segment shows simultaneous verbal-sign training (SV). The last segment shows a probe one week later with no interim training (WK). ▲ denotes days interobserver reliability measures were taken. (From Kotkin et al., 1978, p. 23. Copyright National Society for Mentally Handicapped Children and Adults. Reproduced with permission).

As shown in the figure, the three behaviors formed the multiple baselines when they were measured in the probes during the verbal training (VT) phase, not when they were measured in the first phase (the PB phase), although the procedures in PB and the probes were the same. That is, the multiple-baseline aspect, extending baseline measures on the as yet untrained behaviors was not started until the first training procedure was administered. A more detailed explanation of the phases will clarify this point.

Two training procedures were used in the study; verbal imitation training alone (VT) and simultaneous signing and verbal imitation training (SV). The sign-verbal training always followed the verbal-only training. The pre-baseline procedure required verbal naming on three separate days. After this was completed, VT training was initiated. In VT the experimenter placed a picture in front of the child and named it. If the child imitated the name, he or she was praised and given a piece of food. According to the data in the figures, the multiple-baseline design called for three days of VT on the first name, six days of VT on the second picture, and nine days of VT on the third picture. Thus, the procedure conforming to a multiple-baseline format was contained in the VT condition, not in the PB condition. Baseline for behavior 1 (first word) lasted three days, for behavior 2 (second word) six days, and for behavior 3 (third word) nine days.

When the specified number of training sessions for each word had passed, the second intervention was introduced. At this point, the experimenter provided both the sign and the verbal label for the picture, and the subject was praised and presented with food for correct responses. (The authors do not define correct responses for this phase of training.) The multiple baseline functioned in the following manner. After three days of verbal training, simultaneous sign-verbal training was started for the first word. (This was on the seventh day of the experiment because the first three days had been devoted to pre-baseline.) Meanwhile, the other two words continued to be presented in VT. Three days later, on the ninth day, SV was started on the second word while VT continued on the third word. SV was then initiated on the third word on the twelfth day.

Each training day a probe was administered. The probe consisted of presenting the three pictures to the subject and asking, "What's this?" to elicit a spontaneous naming of the pictures. Recall that this was the pre-baseline procedure and measured the dependent variable in the study. Each picture was presented 20 times during a probe. Correct responses were reinforced. A correct response was defined as a word, a sign, or both. The data in the figure consist of the number of correct responses to the question, "What's this?" in pre-baseline, in the probes during training, and in a final probe a week after training was terminated. Training data are not presented. Both subjects were administered identical treatment except for the words trained. Subject 2 was trained on three words different from those trained for subject 1. Otherwise, the procedures in all phases were the same for the two subjects.

As shown in the figure, neither child produced names for the three pictures in the PB assessment. When VT was initiated only one name was produced spontaneously by subject 1 on the probes. Subject 2 spontaneously named "watermelon" a few times, and "worm" and "tomato" once on a probe. Essentially, spontaneous naming remained at zero level on the probes as it had in pre-baseline. When the simultaneous sign-verbal training was initiated, both subjects increased spontaneous naming to a high level and retained it when tested a week later.

The unusual feature in this study was that the multiple baseline was initiated during the treatment phase of all three behaviors. It is customary, in multiple-baseline studies, to conduct baseline measures on all behaviors involved before treatment (similar to the PB phase in this study). Then treatment is initiated on one of the behaviors, not all behaviors simultaneously. Rather the remaining behaviors continue to be monitored until treated sequentially. In the study by Kotkin et al. (1978), probes for changes in spontaneous naming continued, but imitated naming was already in treatment. Obviously, the VT had only minimal influence on spontaneous naming, so the investigators demonstrated the control essential in a multiple-baseline study. The procedural variation introduced by pursuing the behaviors during treatment was not necessarily inappropriate, just a bit risky in case the treatment proved effective. The study was presented in this chapter partly to demonstrate how investigators may modify basic designs to suit their particular purposes, or when the need arises. If control is demonstrated when a modification is made, the investigator can be complimented on being innovative. Kotkin, Simpson, and DeSanto deserve recognition for their flexibility in design.

We move now to an examination of other components in the Kotkin et al. (1978) experiment from the viewpoint of basics in multiple-baseline designs. It is understood that the standard in our inspection is the ideal design, a form seldom attained in the everyday conduct of research.

Like many other multiple-baseline studies, counterbalancing was not included as a component in the design. Counterbalancing could have been planned for both the three words used for training, and the two training procedures. Of the two, counterbalancng treatments probably would add greater control to the experimental design. The two variables will be discussed separately.

If word order had been counterbalanced each word would have been trained first, second, and third so that all order effects could be cancelled. Controlling for word order would result in a design involving six subjects as illustrated in Table 2.

As suggested earlier, controlling for order of treatments would have strengthened the design even more than accounting for word order. Certainly the data present no evidence that spontaneous naming was influenced by the verbal-only training. Responses on the probes attest to that. One could ask, however, whether the verbal-imitation training affected the children's responses on the probes during sign-verbal training. After all, they had received considerable practice in producing the names before signs were introduced. This practice could influence the way in which the children responded in the second intervention (SV). It would be possible to examine such effects by studying the training data to ascertain the children's performance on the training tasks regardless of performance on the probes. However, one of the selection criteria was ability to imitate the words verbally. From that information one could reasonably assume that the children may have performed well in the verbal-imitation training phase. These speculations could have been put to rest by counterbalancing treatments across children. For example, subject 1 could have received VT first and SV second, whereas subject 2 could have received SV first and VT second. Then, if SV still resulted in more correct spontaneous naming responses, even when it was not preceded by VT, the investigators could be more confident that VT had no influence on performance in SV, or on the probes during SV. Absence of counterbalancing treatments when more than one is administered allows speculation of the presence of variables other than the independent variable which could logically have influenced the results obtained.

One final point should be made regarding the procedures in the Kotkin et al. (1978) study. During the probe presentations on each training day correct responses were reinforced. The investigators' definition of a probe is dif-

Table 2. An example of the permutations necessary in order to control for order effects when three behaviors are studied

Subject	Order of Behaviors			Order of Words[a]		
1	1	2	3	camel	bat	seal
2	1	3	2	camel	seal	bat
3	2	3	1	bat	seal	camel
4	2	1	3	bat	camel	seal
5	3	1	2	seal	camel	bat
6	3	2	1	seal	bat	camel

[a]Words used are from Kotkin et al. (1978).

ferent from the one presented in this book. Generally, a probing procedure is identical to the procedure in baseline assessment. That is, no feedback concerning correctness or incorrectness of responses is provided so as to tap the subject's level of responding aside from training. When consequent events, feedback, follow responses the procedure changes from one of probing to one of training. Feedback is used to cue a subject to the accuracy of the response, providing an opportunity to change it if it is incorrect, or to maintain it if it is correct. Thus, the probes may have provided training data rather than showing how VT and SV affected spontaneous naming.

MULTIPLE-BASELINE ACROSS SETTINGS

A topic of vital interest to interventionists is generalization. Treatment in the clinical setting, or laboratory, may be entirely satisfactory, but for unknown reasons the behavior change is not extended to other settings nor to other individuals. Numerous studies have been conducted exploring variables governing generalization. Multiple-baseline designs can also be used to test generalization, but they are more often used to determine if a treatment is effective in more than one setting. The effect in such studies is akin to a gradual development of generalization.

The number of settings and individuals can vary in the studies, there are no hard and fast rules. It is useful to keep in mind, however, that counterbalancing is as desirable in setting designs as it is in design across behaviors.

Fundamentally, the principles remain the same in all multiple-baseline designs, be they across behaviors, settings, times of day, or other dimensions. Only a few specifics change according to the source of the multiple baseline. In a multiple-baseline design across settings, the same treatment of one behavior is administered to a subject sequentially across different settings. Baseline is taken in all settings initially; then one setting is selected for administering treatment. Baseline continues to be measured in the remaining settings, and when training in the first setting is terminated, it is shifted to the second setting, and so on.

The multiple-baseline design across settings is reminiscent of the procedures used with stutterers after they had learned to control their stuttering in the clinic while continuing to stutter elsewhere. The stutterer would be accompanied to various places, for example, post offices, stores, and restaurants, and requested to use the controls learned in the clinic for speaking fluently. The difference between the multiple-baseline designs across settings and the procedures used to help stutterers to carry over their fluent speech, of course, is that the former is a controlled evaluation of treatment for bringing about a change in a variety of places, and the latter is an uncontrolled, often simultaneous testing procedure applied in all settings at the same time. Both, however, address somewhat similar issues.

If an experimenter were interested in a controlled evaluation of stuttering treatment in a number of settings the following design could be used. The settings might be a post office, a drug store, and a coffee shop. Baseline of stuttering in each setting would be obtained until a stable rate was evident, as defined by the experimenter.

Treatment might consist of a time-out procedure in which the experimenter turns away from the stutterer as soon as disfluency starts. In baseline the experimenter would accompany the stutterer to the three settings, but would not turn away when disfluency occurred as the stutterer spoke. The three settings would be visited in random order during baseline to prevent operation of order effects. For example, on the first day the stutterer and experimenter might go to the post office, drug store, and coffee shop, in that order. On the second baseline day the order might be drug store first, post office second, and coffee shop third. In this way on each baseline day the order would vary from the day before. When baseline stabilized, treatment would begin in setting one, possibly the drug store. Baseline in the other two settings would continue. Treatment in the drug store would be administered for a specific length of time, and when it terminated, treatment would be shifted to the second setting, perhaps the post office. When treatment in the post office setting ended, treatment would begin in the coffee shop setting.

The question in studies of multiple baselines across settings might well be whether a particular treatment is effective in more than one setting. It might also be concerned with determination of the number of settings in which a treatment must be applied before a behavior changes without treatment in a variety of settings. For instance, four settings could be selected and the behavior measured in each before treatment. Treatment is then introduced in the first setting. If the behavior has not changed in the other settings after setting one treatment, the treatment is shifted to the second setting. However, after treatment has been completed in two settings, the behavior may have changed in settings three and four so that treatment need not be administered in them. Questions concerning setting generalization, of course, are less suitable for a multiple-baseline study because the design assumes the independence of the various settings or the multiple-baseline control is lost.

Referring to an earlier statement in this subsection, a variety of parameters would fit into this category of multiple-baseline designs. It is possible to explore behavioral change across different time periods, if these appear relevant. If so, the behavior could be measured, for instance, in the morning, in the afternoon, and in the evening and treatment could be administered in sequence across the three time periods. Individuals could serve a similar purpose, so that behavior would be tested across such categories of people as friends, teachers, and strangers. The multiple-baseline study is designed to explore behavior change across parameters that are relevant for particular behaviors.

In all of the multiple-baseline designs described thus far, the subject has served as his own control. That is, each subject is administered treatment across settings, individuals, and so forth. When behaviors serve as the multiple baseline, the behaviors are still within the subject; that is, they are behaviors that can be studied within one subject. Some multiple-baseline studies, however, do not adhere to the principle that a subject serves as his own control. These designs will be discussed next.

MULTIPLE-BASELINE ACROSS SUBJECTS

Subjects may serve as controls in multiple-baseline studies. An experimenter may select, for example, a number of subjects with similar communication problems. Baseline of the behavior of interest is obtained on all of the subjects. When baseline is stable for all, the first subject is administered treatment as baseline is extended for the other subjects. After treatment of subject 1 has continued for a specified period of time or is completed, subject 2 is started in treatment. Initiation of treatment is sequenced across subjects until all subjects are in treatment. As in multiple-baseline studies across behaviors or settings, the number of subjects in the study may vary according to experimental demands.

Two components in the designs across subjects are different from those in designs using behaviors or settings for control. One difference is that the subject does not serve as his own control in a multiple-baseline design across subjects. Instead, other subjects function as controls. Consequently, one of the components of experimental single-subject designs is modified. Insofar as each subject goes through an A and a B phase only once, replication with another behavior in the same subject, or across another setting with the same subject does not occur. Absence of a replication within each subject results in shifting control to others.

Because a number of subjects are used to achieve control, subject characteristics take on greater importance. If the subjects differ from each other, the variability might be reflected in the results of the manipulation. Imagine, for example, that one subject performs differently from the others in treatment. Naturally, the difference could be caused by a number of variables; but a strong suspect among them is subject characteristics. The suspicion arises because other components of the experiment are constant.

An explanation is sought where variation is found, and subject characteristics form a reasonable explanation. Needless to say, subject characteristics do not always serve to confound results; they simply offer the possibility if control is shifted from within a single subject to others who might differ from each other. The factors making subjects unlike could potentially account for differences in performance.

Another difference between the multiple-baseline design across subjects and other multiple-baseline designs is that counterbalancing is not a component in the design across subject. This is not because investigators neglect to employ counterbalancing; no consideration need be given to it. Not only is it unnecessary, it is impossible to counterbalance in a design across subjects.

An example of a multiple-baseline design across subjects is found in a study conducted by Tucker and Berry (1980). The study was designed to evaluate the effectiveness of a comprehensive instructional package for teaching mentally retarded hearing-impaired subjects to put on their hearing aids. Generalization to other environments was also assessed in the study. The report described three experiments involving hearing aids, but for the purpose of illustrating a multiple-baseline design across subjects, only the first part of the first experiment is described. Detailed procedural information is not included.

Generally, the investigators developed a 10-component program starting with picking up the hearing aid, learning to insert it into the pocket of a shirt, inserting the ear mold into the ear, turning the aid on, and setting the gain control. The instructional package also contained several levels of instructions for training the subjects to complete each step. Thus, the independent variable (instructional package) consisted of a complex program with many parts, not just one variable. The dependent variable consisted of following the step-by-step procedure for putting on a hearing aid without instructions or assistance from a trainer. The program had been developed from observations and pilot tests on other individuals in the institution.

Although six subjects were studied, only three were reported in the first experiment. The subjects were severely multihandicapped residents at an institution for the mentally and physically handicapped ranging in age from 19.9 to 22.3 years. A multiple-baseline design across three subjects was used to explore the effectiveness of the training program in teaching subjects to put on their hearing aids. The design, without the generalization component, is shown in Figure 14. Data consisted of percentage of program steps completed correctly without any assistance from the trainer. Baseline consisted of addressing the subject by name and instructing the subject to "Please put on your hearing aid." After a baseline of four sessions, subject 1, Susan, was started in training. Baseline for Tom, subject 2, consisted of seven

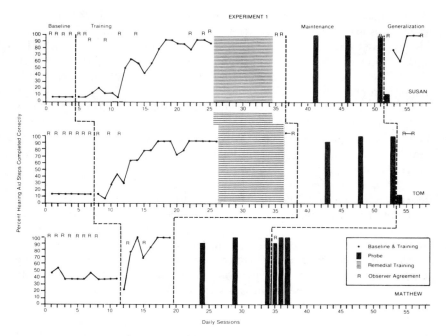

Figure 14. Percentage of hearing aid steps completed correctly without trainer assistance for Susan, Tom, and Matthew. The shaded area for Susan and Tom represents the period of time required for remedial training on the program step in which their behavior was deficient. *Connected dots* represent performance in the training setting. *Vertical bars* represent maintenance and generalization probe behavior. The *R* represents the level of reliability agreement for a given session. (From Tucker and Berry, 1980, p. 72. Copyright by Society for the Experimental Analysis of Behavior, Inc. Reproduced with permission).

sessions, and subject 3, Matthew, continued in baseline for 11 sessions before entering the training program. The design, therefore, was a multiple-baseline design across the three subjects for experiment 1.

As mentioned, only data on acquisition were selected for presentation in Figure 14. Baselines for subjects 1 and 2 were lower than for subject 3. Acquisition data show differences, also, and might have been related to differences in baseline performance. In addition to the difference in baseline, Susan and Tom required extra remedial instruction and more training sessions than Matthew, who completed training in about half as many sessions. Nevertheless, the program effectively trained all three subjects to put on their hearing aids.

The reason for the difference in performance between Matthew and the other two subjects is not apparent. Comprehensive descriptions of the subjects were not included, but two differences can be identified, regarding auditory performance. Matthew had a conductive loss whereas the other two had sensorineural losses; and Matthew wore a bone-conduction hearing aid, whereas the other two wore air-conduction hearing aids. Possibly, Matthew heard and comprehended instructions with greater ease than did the other two subjects. Matthew, with better baseline performance and a different kind of hearing loss, may not have been the ideal control for the other two subjects. They were too unlike.

The doubt concerning Matthew in no way invalidates the results of the study; it was raised because a design using subjects as a multiple baseline is more vulnerable to confounds than designs in which subjects can serve as their own controls. Problems may arise in these studies that can be averted by using designs more compatible with the rationale behind single-subject experimental designs, or careful matching of subjects. In any case, using designs across subjects should alert the investigator to attending to more details associated with subject characteristics. Matching subjects on as many relevant characteristics as possible might help to alleviate sources of variability.

MULTIPLE-BASELINE ACROSS GROUPS

Another version of the multiple baseline design across subjects is the multiple-baseline across groups. The groups frequently consist of entire classrooms. In these studies baseline is measured in more than one classroom. After a number of sessions in baseline, treatment is administered to classroom 1. The remaining classrooms are continued in baseline. After a specified number of sessions, treatment is administered to the second classroom, while the third continues in baseline for additional sessions. Thus, each classroom serves as a control to demonstrate that performance of the entire class changes only when intervention is initiated. Needless to say, the multiple-baseline design across groups is even further removed from the concept of subjects serving as their own controls.

ISSUES IN MULTIPLE-BASELINE DESIGNS

It is generally acknowledged that multiple baseline designs are weaker in controls than A-B-A-B designs (Hersen and Barlow, 1976; Kratochwill, 1978). This is because replication, even when two behaviors of a single subject are studied, occurs on different behaviors rather than on the same behavior. In the case of multiple-baseline designs across settings, the settings differ. And, of course, as already mentioned, control shifts further away from the subject himself in multiple-baseline designs across subjects and groups. Essentially, only the A-B-A-B design conforms precisely to a definition of within-subject control.

Number of Replications

Discussion has centered on how many replications are necessary in multiple-baseline studies to demonstrate experimental control, and thereby, treatment effectiveness. For greater confidence in results suggestions range between at least three (Wolf and Risley, 1971) and four behaviors (Kazdin and Kopel, 1975; Hersen and Barlow 1976), although two might sometimes be considered sufficient. As pointed out earlier, however, the more behaviors (and settings) studied, the greater the risk of order effects; and controlling for order effects requires a greater number of subjects. Moreover, the more replications, the longer the baselines for the untreated behaviors. That is, the third and fourth behaviors would have to continue for extended periods. Conceivably, the fourth behavior could remain in baseline for many sessions or many days. A lengthy baseline could prove disadvantageous in a number of ways. It could, possibly, present ethical or social problems if the behaviors consisted of responses needing treatment as soon as possible. Conversely, continual sampling of a behavior over a long period may precipitate changes in that behavior due to the continuous measurement, so that patterns or trends appear in baseline, or variability ensues. An experimenter must balance these factors carefully in deciding how many baselines to include in one study.

Baseline Procedures

There are no established rules about measuring the behaviors continued in baseline during sequential treatment of several others. Assuredly, the ideal procedure is to take baseline measurements on the untreated behaviors each time treatment is administered on the behavior or behaviors currently in the intervention phase. This would entail measures of the untreated behaviors in each training session. Examination of studies reported in the literature revealed that practices differ considerably among investigators. In the Bennett (1974) study, for instance, the second sound was probed only once between baseline and initiation of training, not in each session while the first sound was being trained. In contrast, a probe of the untrained words was administered in each training session in the Kotkin, Simpson, and DeSanto (1978) study. At times, baseline for the untreated behaviors is obtained intermittently, perhaps in every third or fourth training session. Intermittent measures may be less efficient in terms of complying to the demands of multiple-baseline designs, but they may be more practical when lengthy baselines are required in studies of multiple baselines.

Another issue for consideration in multiple-baseline studies is determining when treatment should be initiated for each baseline. Assume that four behaviors (or four settings, subjects, or groups) are involved in the multiple-baseline design. The experimenter must decide when training on the second, third, and fourth behaviors should begin. Here, also, practice varies considerably among investigators, and reasons for choices are seldom disclosed in reports in the literature. Ideally, it is best to defer training on behavior 2 until training on behavior 1 has been completed; and behavior 3 should not be started in treatment until training on behavior 2 has terminated. Similarly, behavior 4 is not adminstered treatment until training on behavior 3 has been completed. Such sequencing would demonstrate maximum control because in each case training would have been completed, and yet the behavior next in line would not have changed during the entire period. Obviously, such procedures could prolong a study indefinitely, particularly when more than two baselines are involved, and might create problems in maintaining stability on the untreated baselines. For this reason, and undoubtedly others, the criterion that training of one behavior must be completed before treatment is started on the next is seldom applied. Generally, experimenters specify a number of days, or sessions, for each untreated baseline, basing initiation of training on passage of time. For example, training on behavior 2 may be initiated when behavior 1 has been in training for three days, and behavior 3 is started in training when an additional three days have passed, and so on. Usually equal amounts of time for each baseline are programmed. This procedure was followed in the Kotkin et al. (1978) study and the Tucker and Berry (1980) study. In the former study, three days separated initiation of training for words 2 and 3, and in the latter, it appeared that four-day intervals were used across subjects. On the other hand, in Bennett's (1974) study, training on behavior 2 was not initiated until criterion on behavior 1 had been reached. The rationale for initiation of training in multiple-baseline studies is not always clear, and is probably more perplexing when initiations are unevenly spaced as in a study of adjective and adverb training in hearing-impaired and aphasic children (Heward and Eachus, 1979). The investigators did not report how many baseline sessions were required for the three behaviors studied, or the reasons for their choice. From their data it appeared that 27 days of baseline were taken on behavior 2, but only 15 days on behavior 3. Irrespective of prior decisions, one important factor overrides any others regarding baseline length. Treatment should not be initiated if the baseline evidences instability.

Behavioral Covariance

One of the advantages of multiple-baseline designs, according to Kazdin (1973), Kratochwill (1978), and Hersen and Barlow (1976), is that the designs allow simultaneous measurement of more than one target behavior. This implies that they resemble naturalistic conditions more than A-B-A-B designs in which only one target behavior is measured. Also, it is said, measurement of more than one behavior allows observation of changes in behavior other than the target behavior receiving treatment. In turn, examination of relationships between the behaviors is possible. Undoubtedly, the point is well made; examination of several behaviors during treatment of one may reveal if they are covariant. The idea, however, seems contrary to the concept in the methodology of multiple-baseline designs. Supposedly, the behaviors are selected for their independence from each other. Should the untreated behaviors change during treatment of another, multiple-baseline control would be lost. In this case, the experimenter would hesitate before drawing conclusions about the effectiveness of the training variable on the target behavior. Conclusions about relationships between the other behaviors being measured would be much less certain.

Extraneous Variable Effects

Another conflicting assumption in multiple-baseline designs has been examined by Kazdin and Kopel (1975). The rationale behind multiple-baseline designs is that the influence of extraneous variables on behavior can be ruled out if behavior changes only when treatment is administered. If extraneous events were operating on the behavior during treatment, they would also be operating on the untreated behaviors. If the as yet untreated behaviors remained unchanged, then extraneous variables are not confounding treatment. But, as Kazdin and Kopel (1975) point out, the design appears based on two conflicting assumptions about extraneous variables. It assumes that extraneous variables will affect all behaviors, whereas treatment variables will affect only the specific behavior being treated. The authors observe that it is inconsistent to assume that certain types of events (extraneous variables) have generalized effects and other kinds of events (treatment) have specific effects. It is more reasonable to assume that both types of events can have both kinds of effects. More to the point, extraneous events can influence specific behaviors as readily as treatment, and treatment may effect changes in untreated behaviors. Investigators are reminded that if intervention of one behavior is correlated with changes in other behaviors in the multiple baseline as well, it is not possible to attribute the changes either to treatment or to extraneous variables, because one or both could have been responsible.

When results are clear and the multiple baseline holds, investigators need not be concerned about the problem. Nonetheless, to minimize confounding, Kazdin and Kopel (1975) offer three recommendations. They suggest 1) selecting baselines that are as independent as possible, 2) using several, instead of a few, baselines, and 3) designing a reversal phase for one of the behaviors. The first recommendation has already been discussed. The reason for the second recommendation is that when several behaviors are used, one or two may change, but behaviors less closely associated with the behavior in treatment may remain unchanged. Finally, a reversal will provide a controlled demonstration that the treatment was responsible for changes in the behavior treated.

SUMMARY

The multiple-baseline study consists, basically, of an A-B design replicated across behaviors, settings, subjects, or groups. In a two-baseline study, baseline is measured for both. When treatment is introduced for the first baseline, the second remains in baseline measurement. The second baseline receives treatment only after a specified period of treatment has been completed for the first baseline. Several forms of multiple-baseline designs are available and can be selected at the experimenter's discretion.

Multiple-baseline designs are an excellent alternative to A-B-A-B designs when the behaviors to be treated are not amenable to extinction or reversal. Although not as strong a design as an A-B-A-B, the multiple-baseline design nevertheless allows a broader view of replication possibilities because different behaviors, settings, and individuals are involved in the designs.

Two assumptions must be made in use of multiple-baseline designs: 1) the baselines are independent of each other, and 2) the same treatment is applicable to each baseline. These assumptions are critical to designs across behaviors and settings, but the first assumption is less crucial across subjects and groups.

Length of phases, number of measurements of each untreated baseline, and timing of treatment initiation are issues that have not been solved. Decisions regarding these factors are based on the behaviors and treatments investigated. It has been recommended that a three- or four-baseline design provides strong evidence of treatment effectiveness.

In this book the A-B-A-B and multiple-baseline have been treated as basic designs in within-subject experimental studies. This viewpoint is justified partly on the basis of frequency of use in studies. The A-B-A-B and multiple-baseline designs predominate behavioral and communicative disorders research in single-subject studies. Other designs are available, but thus far their application in behavior research is minimal, and almost nonexistent in the communicative disorders literature. There is another reason for the emphasis on A-B-A-B and multiple-baseline designs. Several of the newer designs appearing in the behavioral research literature share many features with the A-B-A-B and multiple-baseline designs. In fact, some could rightfully be described as modifications of the basic designs. Therefore, if the basic designs are understood, the alternative designs should be more comprehensible. Hopefully, this reasoning bears out in the presentation of alternative designs in Chapter 6. They are treated briefly in comparison to the discussions of the A-B-A-B and multiple-baseline designs. This is necessary because information on their usefulness is lacking until additional studies have been completed. Before the shift to discussion of the recently introduced designs, however, a chapter devoted to a detailed explanation of the conditions or phases in A-B-A-B and multiple-baseline designs is presented. Emphasis in the next chapter, therefore, is placed on criteria to be met in each experimental phase to demonstrate experimental control and treatment effects.

Criteria for Evaluating Data for Treatment Effectiveness

4

In the first three chapters the rationale for within-subject designs and basic components of A-B-A-B and multiple-baseline designs are described. In this chapter, criteria for evaluating treatment effectiveness regardless of study design are explored. Evaluation of treatment effectiveness is not restricted to evaluation of the data within individual studies. Indeed, equally important in experimental analysis research is evaluation of data across studies in relation to clinical and social importance for populations represented by the subjects and disorders examined in individual studies.

Criteria may be placed, then, into three broad categories. Category one includes factors to be considered in evaluating effectiveness of treatment within an individual study. Some overlap with category one occurs in the factors evaluated in category two, because within this category generality is explored in reference to replications within and across studies. The third category includes factors to be weighed in terms of clinical and social validity and importance, that is, degree of generality to populations with similar and different disorders.

Each category is discussed individually, recognizing the overlap between categories. The discussion is preceded, however, by an overview of the kind of data obtained and data analysis procedures used to evaluate treatment effectiveness.

MEASUREMENT AND DATA ANALYSIS

Intervention research, which of course is what single-subject experimental research is about, seldom uses any form of indirect measurement. It is behavioral research and so it is behavior that is measured. In psychotherapy research, indirect measures sometimes constitute the dependent variable, as in responses to projective or personality tests, or self-reports of behavior. Similar measures may be employed occasionally in communicative disorders research, but they are less prevalent than in psychology. Not that all measures in communicative disorders studies are direct observations of the behavior of interest. For example, auditory memory is customarily studied indirectly. Responses in these studies may be motor, as in button presses, written, or verbal, in which the subject verbally reproduces items in sequences as they were presented either visually or auditorially. The responses and response patterns in these studies are interpreted as representing what the subject remembers of the stimuli presented. But this is not a direct measurement of ''memory'' because memory is an abstract concept that cannot be measured directly.

In experimental analysis of behavior designs, the preference is to study the target behavior directly. If mathematics is explored, the subject's ability to complete problems may constitute the dependent variable. In communicative disorders research, if a change in voice is the target in treatment, the dependent variable is a measure of voice parameters; if language is the target, the aspects of language to be manipulated are measured directly, for example, plurals or auxiliary verbs. Recently, however, cognition has been introduced as an important research target in communicative disorders. Because cognition is also an abstract target that cannot be measured directly, but must be inferred from the occurrence of other behaviors, it poses problems for studies intended to measure the target behavior directly. Of course, operational definitions of cognition may serve this purpose adequately in studies. For example, cognition may be defined as ability to sort animal pictures from pictures of furniture and to place them in appropriate piles. The behavior studied is sorting behavior, but the experimenter may define the sorting behavior as one form of cognition. These indirect measures may be used by communicative disorders researchers, but the most common measures in experimental analysis of behavior research is counting the actual occurrence of the behavior itself. If the behavior is to be measured directly it must: 1) be specified clearly, 2) be observable, 3) be public, and 4) be replicable.

The behavior itself may be measured in a number of ways. The most frequent is simply occurrence or nonoccurrence of the response over a specified time period as in counting occurrence of stuttering in a 10-minute period in which the subject is reading aloud. The experimenter adopts a time period conforming closely and realistically to the natural occurrence of the behavior. To illustrate with an extreme example, one would not count occurrence of stuttering over a 24-hour period because people seldom read for 24 hours straight. Ten minutes, on the other hand, is not only a plausible time period, but a natural and reasonable one. The experimenter makes the decision regarding the response to be measured and the period in which it is to be measured based on the kind of behavior studied and conditions under which measurements will be made.

The basic principle in selecting the behavior for measurement and the occasion and condition under which it will be measured is that it should be one that gives the most accurate accounting. For instance, measuring the number of word repetitions would not provide clear information about an aphasic's language problem. It is important to pick a response that fits the behavior to be treated.

Unit of Measurement

Originally in experimental analysis research, rate of responding across units of time was the predominant measure. Each response was recorded and the dependent variable was defined as a change in the rate of the response as a function of the independent variable over time. Rate is still the basic measure, but it may be modified to conform to a particular response studied. Thus, the experimenter may present the number of responses, the frequency of a response, or the percentage of responses from a total number of responses, all over specified time segments. Depending on the study procedures, responses may be counted on a trial-by-trial basis, or alternatively, over specified time intervals. If the response requires use of paper and pencil, as in completing math problems, the dependent variable may be rate (number of problems completed in a particular time interval), but also the accuracy of the answers for the problems completed. Thus, although basically some form of rate is involved in measurement, other parameters may be used if rate is not the most appropriate. Nonetheless, the basic datum is change in number, frequency, percentage of a specified behavior over time both when the independent variable is absent and when it is present. Parsonson and Baer (1978) have summarized the four forms data may take (p. 115):

> They may be expressed in terms of *frequency of occurrence,* usually the proportion of recording intervals in which the target behavior occurred at least once:
>
> $$\frac{\text{intervals in which response occurred}}{\text{total intervals available}} \times \frac{100}{1}$$
>
> *rate of occurrence,* the ratio of the number of times the target behavior occurred per unit of observation time:
>
> $$\frac{\text{number of responses}}{\text{time unit}}$$

duration of occurrence, the total time of occurrence of the behavior as a proportion of the total observation time:

$$\frac{\text{time of behavior}}{\text{time of observation}} \times \frac{100}{1}$$

or *percentage of responses,* usually expressed as the proportion of time the behavior occurs per opportunity:

$$\frac{\text{number of responses}}{\text{number of opportunities}} \times \frac{100}{1}$$

These forms are appropriate for most communicative disorders research in which treatment is the independent variable. Frequency of occurrence, for example, could be used in measuring the number of intervals in which a child addresses a question to a peer in six 10-minute intervals during an hour-long play period in a language group. Rate of occurrence is a common measure in communicative disorders, as in recording the number of disfluencies within a 30-minute monologue. Duration of occurrence is an appropriate measure when the length of time a child attends to a task is measured during a 40-minute classroom period. Articulation of correct sounds lends itself well to measures involving percentages of responses. If a child is provided with 100 trials in which to produce a target sound and produces it correctly on 20 of them, the data can be presented in the form of percentage correct in 100 opportunities, or 20% correct responses. Unit of measurement is not restricted to the four offered by Parsonson and Baer (1978), but they predominate in the data presented in single-subject experimental designs.

At times experimenters prefer to group their data in some way, particularly when variability is obvious and it is difficult to evaluate the effect of treatment. Grouping data may also be used when data points number too many to place comfortably on one graph. Collapsing the data may take the form of averaging the data from 2, 3, 4, or more sessions.

Even though this practice is acceptable, it strays from the principle of repeated measures in within-subject designs. Using averages may smooth out the variability visually, but does not eliminate it. If averaged data lulls the experimenter or reader into ignoring the variability, the purpose of repeated measurement may be defeated. One of the advantages of using repeated measures is that it reveals variability when it is present before and during intervention so that causes for the variability can be explored experimentally. When averaged data obscure the actual form of the behavior over time a chance to pursue causes may be missed. As Hersen and Barlow (1976) suggest, most investigators prefer to present all the data from the course of the study so that intra- and intersubject variability can be examined. In this way, each investigator studying the data is free to draw his or her own conclusions regarding importance of the variability to the treatment studied.

It was mentioned previously that in the last few years single-subject investigators have been encouraged to use statistics to determine the significance of their treatment to a disorder. Opinion on the topic is divided (Gentile, Roden, and Klein, 1972; Michael, 1974a and b; Carver, 1978; Johnston and Pennypacker, 1980). Perhaps the strongest argument against the use of statistics is that if statistics are necessary to tease out the effect of a treatment, the treatment is not apt to be considered clinically relevant. More will be said about this issue later in the chapter. For a comprehensive review of the pros and cons, the following references are useful: Edgington, 1967; Hartmann, 1974; Jones, Vaught, and Weinrott, 1977; Jones, Weinrott, and Vaught, 1978; Kazdin, 1975b, 1976, 1978; Kratochwill, 1978; Michael, 1974a and b; and Thoresen and Elashoff, 1974).

Conservative investigators continue to support use of visual displays in graphs in which responses are depicted as they actually occur over a period of time. Parsonson and Baer (1978) refer to this as graphic analysis.

Form of Data Analysis

Graphed data are primary data, not data that have been smoothed or treated in some way so that they are removed from close contact with the behavior being manipulated. Emphasis is on demonstrating direct and individualized experimental control in within-subject research designs. This can be demonstrated best by presenting direct and individualized data. As Parsonson and Baer (1978) pointed out, "The behavior of the subject(s) controls the pace and procedures which are continuously available to the experimenter who graphed after each session" (p. 109). They continue by suggesting that this form of data analysis allows the experimenter to modify or change procedures if the data indicate need for changes. This flexibility is an advantage of repeated measures designs in which the behavior is continuously monitored (Johnston and Pennypacker, 1980). In truth this flexibility has not been demonstrated often in the published literature, and as far as communicative disorders research is concerned, studies that change in midstream are scarce. Whether this reluctance is due to publication standards, investigator reluctance to report such studies, or nonoccurrence is unclear.

Aside from flexibility within a study, direct measurement of the ongoing target behavior undoubtedly serves to reveal any variability that occurs. The course of treatment is seldom smooth or linear, as clinicians can testify. In a before-and-after study the behavioral course cannot be examined, so little information can be obtained on when the treatment bogs down or results in an abrupt change in the right direction. Conversely, repeated measures are designed for the purpose of clearly showing all changes. Such revelations should be helpful to the experimenter later when another study is designed to examine some aspect of the variability found in the first study. Moreover, for clinicians who would apply the procedures in treating a client, the information allows them to expect differences in progress of training, to predict the course of progress. And this, in turn, could prevent abandonment of a treatment prematurely. All other considerations aside, Parsonson and Baer (1978) make the point that ''. . . experimental designs and forms of data analysis that do not isolate researchers from direct, continuing contact with their subject matter, or smooth out interesting variations in performance, may broaden the scope of scientific discovery.'' (p. 109). Obviously they do not favor averaging or statistical analysis of data. We tend to agree with this stand, but recognize reasons for the development of statistics amenable to handling time-series designs. Perhaps one reason for statistical evaluation is that some behaviors under study are more complex. However, the major reason may lie in designs that are increasingly popular in special education and education. The designs employ groups of subjects, several ex- perimenters, some less trained that others, and settings differing from each other in a number of ways. Naturally all these variables can function to obscure treatment effects partially, so that only weak effects are found. Desir- ing to determine what these weak effects may mean, the experimenter turns to an instrument that will handle variation and reveal the operation of the treatment. The designs and data analyses in these cases are removed from the purpose of single-subject experimental designs.

Be that as it may, the discussion now returns to graphic analysis. To reiterate, experiments in applied behavior analysis are composed of two basic components, an A and a B, arranged in different combinations. Further, they are interrupted time-series designs in which observations of the dependent variable are made when the independent variable is absent (A), and when it is present in the treatment (B) or intervention phase of the study.

Recording of data may be made across any segment of time selected by the experimenter. It could be across minutes, hours, sessions, days, weeks, and so forth. As already explained, the data may be presented in terms of fre- quency, rate, duration, or percentage. It has often been proposed that the graph in which data are exhibited should be so clear that a text explaining the data is superfluous. Data are usually displayed over time and across condi- tions.

EVALUATION CRITERIA WITHIN STUDIES

Furlong and Wampold (1981) suggest that four basic questions need to be answered in making visual inferences of treatment effectiveness. The viewer should determine if: 1) the data are reliable, 2) the behavior was altered when the intervention was administered, 3) the change observed was important or meaningful, and 4) the results are generalizable to other individuals. The first two questions refer to form of the data within a study and the last two relate to evaluation across studies as well as social validation. The authors present a visual analysis checklist for evaluating treatment effects.

Evaluation of treatment effects within an individual study is possible by visually comparing the data points in the A phases and the B phases. Aspects to consider in comparison is the next topic and is presented in this section. Briefly, they include: 1) stability of baseline, 2) variability within phases, 3) variability between phases, 4) overlap between scores of adjacent phases, 5) number of data points in each phase, 6) changes in trends within phases, 7) changes in trends between adjacent phases, 8) changes in level between phases, 9) analysis of data across similar phases, and 10) evaluation of overall patterns of the data (Parsonson and Baer, 1978). These factors are discussed individually and in combination under different subheadings.

Baseline

Before discussing baseline criteria specifically, it may be helpful to define three parameters important to data or graphs presented visually. These parameters are used to evaluate the adequacy of the baseline, to compare performance between the baseline phase (A) and the treatment phase (B) and, in an A-B-A design, between treatment (B) and return to baseline (A). If an A-B-A-B design is used one more comparison is possible between the final A and B phases.

The three parameters to be considered include: 1) the trend in the data, 2) the level at which the behavior is occurring according to the data, and 3) the slope in the data pattern. The three parameters are inherent in the 10 aspects mentioned in the previous paragraphs.

Trend   The effectiveness of the independent variable is measured by comparing the direction of the behavior before treatment and after treatment is administered. The three directions the behavior may take include 1) an increase in the occurrence of the behavior, 2) a decrease in the occurrence of the behavior, and 3) no change in occurrence.

Usually an increase involves a behavior defined as desirable by the experimenter and occurs at a low rate before treatment. Hopefully, the treatment will function to increase rate of occurrence. A decrease, on the other hand, involves a high rate of occurrence of a behavior customarily defined by the experimenter as undesirable. Examples of each might be increases in rate of an inflectional rise at the end of questions, and a decrease of words per minute for a clutterer. Thus, what is sought is evidence of a decisive increase or decrease in rate during treatment. The standard against which rate changes are measured is, first of all, baseline.

To establish a believable standard, the behavior must be measured a sufficient number of times to establish that it is not changing before treatment.

It has been recommended that a minimum of three measures are necessary to demonstrate stability. If the rate of occurrence of the behavior is changing from one measurement to the next, stability has not been established and the standard for comparison is unclear. In such cases, it is best to continue measurement of the behavior until the changes cease or are confined within reasonable bounds.

There are several trends that must be considered as precluding introduction of treatment. First, if the treatment is expected to effect an increase, the behavior in baseline cannot show a trend of increasing rate of occurrence. This trend is illustrated in Figure 15a. This increase is unacceptable because if treatment is introduced during an increasing trend it is not possible to attribute continued increases in rate of occurrence to the treatment. Possibly, the behavior would have continued to increase if baseline sessions had been continued and the increase would be similar to the one observed in treatment.

For a treatment designed to increase occurrence of behavior, a decreasing trend in baseline is more acceptable, as shown in Figure 15b. Introduction of treatment when rate is decreasing before treatment allows a dramatic demonstration of treatment effectiveness if the direction of the trend is sharply altered when treatment is introduced.

The reverse criterion holds if the behavior is one occurring at a high rate before treatment and is expected to decrease with treatment as illustrated in Figure 16. In the first case (Figure 16a) a decrease is occurring before treatment, so if treatment is introduced at this point it would not be possible to attribute a continued rate reduction to treatment. But in Figure 16b, introduction of treatment with a resultant rate reduction would provide strong

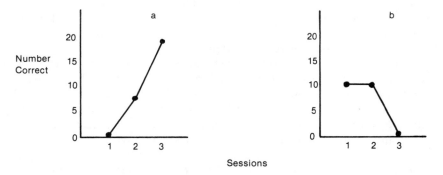

Figure 15. Inappropriate *(a)* and appropriate *(b)* trends in baseline. An increase in rate in baseline before application of treatment expected to effect an increase is an inappropriate trend. A decrease in rate in baseline before application of treatment which is expected to effect an increase is an appropriate trend.

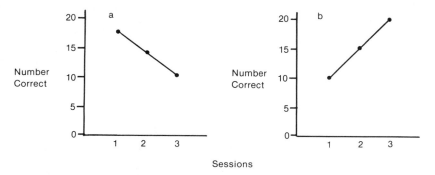

Figure 16. Examples of inappropriate *(a)* and appropriate *(b)* trends in baseline when treatment is expected to effect a decrease in rate of a behavior.

evidence of treatment effectiveness because the trend was reversed in treatment.

Presumably, investigators are likely to be most comfortable with the stable baseline. A trend in either direction may indicate that the behavior is unstable, varying, perhaps unpredictably. The experimenter could not be positive that the next data point would show a trend continuing in the direction of the first three data points, or if it would show a return to the position of the first data point. Assuredly, three stable data points could be followed by a fourth that deviated from the stable pattern, but an unvarying pattern is more comforting than a varying one. Perhaps the best way to state this principle is that baselines showing trends are less predictable than baselines showing little change over measures, even when the change is in the opposite direction from the direction expected during treatment.

A stable baseline refers to repeated measures of the behavior with little variation in occurrence from one measure to the next. Stability is illustrated in the Figure 17, below. Baselines in the figure are ideal, of course, because they show no variation, an unusual event in human behavior. Nevertheless, they make the point. If the behavior is occurring at the same low rate in three measurements, it is safe to introduce treatment to increase the rate. By the same token, if the behavior does not vary from the initial high rate over three baseline measurements, the experimenter can confidently introduce treatment to decrease rate.

Unfortunately, as is obvious to anyone working with disordered clients with communicative problems, not all behaviors occur at consistently low or high rates over time. More commonly, frequency varies, or the behavior is emitted inconsistently. For example, an aphasic client may sometimes produce a particular grammatical structure correctly and at times not produce the structure at all, although the stimulus conditions are the same on both occa-

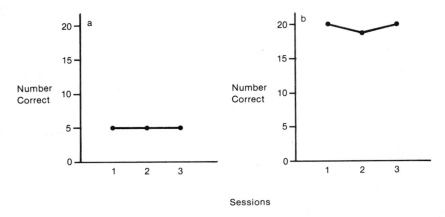

Figure 17. Examples of ideal baseline when an increase in rate is expected *(a)* and a decrease is expected *(b)*.

sions. Misarticulating children will do the same with error sounds. The sounds may be produced correctly in some words and incorrectly in others. An investigator wishing to explore communicative disorders must be prepared to encounter such variability.

If the behavior measured in baseline varies from one measurement period to another, the experimenter has several options for defining an adequate baseline. First, it is possible to set limits as to amount of variability to be tolerated. The amount selected will depend on the behavior studied. At one time variability within a range of 5% to 10% was recommended (Sidman, 1960; Hersen and Barlow, 1976), but investigators no longer insist on these limits, allowing greater flexibility. This is apparent in several studies reported in this text. A certain amount of variability is unavoidable if treatment studies are to be conducted, but it is necessary to keep in mind that baseline is the standard against which treatment effects are measured. If baseline varies too much, changes due to treatment cannot be separated from natural variability of the behavior without treatment.

Another option available to the investigator when variability is apparent is to extend baseline measures to determine whether a pattern is discernible in the variation. That is to say, the investigator examines the rate alternations over a number of measures to ascertain if the low and high rates reveal a cyclical or regular pattern. An example of a pattern in baseline is presented in Figure 18. If the treatment phase reveals a disruption of the pattern or a shift of the pattern up or down, then treatment effects can be demonstrated.

The most reasonable and safest option for handling variability in baseline is to continue baseline measures until stability is established. The

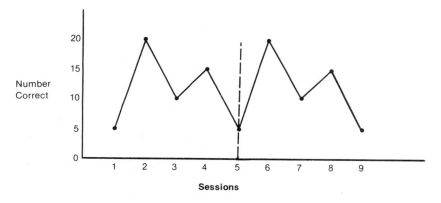

Figure 18. An example of a systematic pattern of variation in baseline.

suggestion for three measures is the minimal number; it is not uncommon to find extended baselines for behaviors. As in all cases, the degree to which a baseline is continued past the minimum three measures depends on several factors: 1) how crucial it is to begin treatment because the behavior cannot be allowed to continue indefinitely; 2) whether the investigator, from past experience with the disorder, has any expectation that the behavior will stabilize; and 3) whether extended measurement of the behavior will in itself function to change the behavior as in practice effects. These and other considerations peculiar to specific disorders will influence the way in which an experimenter handles baseline variability. If possible, continuing baseline until stability is achieved would appear to be the best choice because it conforms to requirements of within-subject designs in which the subject serves as his own control.

Of course, there is always the possibility that, regardless of what the experimenter does, variability continues. In that case, it is better to abandon that particular study than to introduce treatment. (Unless the treatment itself is expected to reduce variability.) More is to be gained by designing another study to explore other behaviors, or better still, to design a study to investigate variables responsible for the baseline variability. Before presenting examples of studies to demonstrate the points made about baseline criteria, a few additional suggestions to strengthen baseline measures may be helpful.

Partly to control for the natural variability found in many communicative behaviors and partly to eliminate the effect of any extraneous variables on the baseline performance, it is recommended that baseline be measured over several sessions or days rather than in one session. If the behavior is measured on different occasions, and it does not vary, the experimenter will have demonstrated stability irrespective of other variables that may be influencing the behavior. Likewise, if the behavior is measured over several days and it remains stable, the experimenter has demonstrated that any extraneous variables present on day one could not have been responsible for the baseline results because on day two and three the results were the same, although other variables may have been present. For instance, it is possible that on day one the subject has a stomachache, which could influence his responses in baseline. To rule out this possible confounding variable, the measure is made again on another day when the subject is physically well. If the same results are obtained on both days, the confounding effect of the stomachache can be ruled out.

It is also important that the conditions under which baseline is measured be kept as constant as possible. Baseline can be affected if the experimenter is changed from one measure to another, or the location is shifted. As in the treatment phase of a study, changes in conditions can influence results so that if variability in baseline is observed, it would be difficult to identify the cause.

Baseline measures are pretreatment measures of the natural occurrence of a behavior and can at times become lengthy. Usually, the experimenter attempts to remain as aloof as possible during baseline, keeping the situation as similar as possible from one occasion to the next. It is important, however, to prevent fatigue, boredom, inattention, or restlessness from influencing the subject's performance. To avoid the influence of these variables, the experimenter can schedule reasonably short sessions or can schedule social or tangible presentations of encouragement in between administration of baseline measures. In language studies, for instance, if a particular grammatical structure is tested, and the subject is emitting the structure at a low rate or not at all, the experimenter may insert language items known to the subject at specified intervals. When these structures are produced by the subject appropriate praise can be presented by the experimenter. Frequently experimenters, at the end of each baseline session, will present the subject with a token of appreciation for participating in the session. Problems with keeping the subject on task in baseline are more frequent when children serve as subjects, but they occur with adults as well if unreasonable demands are placed on them.

Slope   The trend of the data is not the only aspect to be considered in determining adequacy of the baseline. The degree of slope in the trend will indicate how strong the trend is. If there is a pronounced slope in the trend, it is stronger evidence that the behavior is changing than if the slope is a gentle one. The two kinds of slopes are illustrated in Figure 19. The notion of slope is more pertinent to evaluation of treatment effects in comparing the data between the A and B phases of the study. Nevertheless, slope should be used in baseline as well to make decisions concerning the power of a trend and to

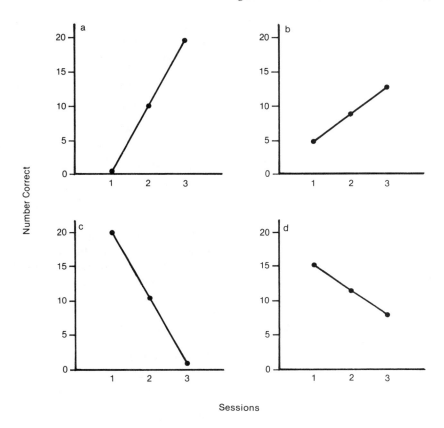

Figure 19. Examples of degrees of slope in trends during baseline. Pronounced slopes are illustrated in *a* and *c* and gentle slopes in *b* and *d*.

determine whether by extending the baseline a plateau will be reached indicating that stability had been achieved.

Level   The final factor contributing to decisions regarding baseline adequacy is the level at which the behavior is occurring before treatment. Obviously, if the behavior is one that the experimenter hopes will increase with treatment, it cannot be occurring at a high rate during pretreatment measures. Conversely, if the behavior is one that needs to be reduced in occurrence, baseline data must demonstrate that it is occurring at a reasonably high rate before treatment. Figure 20 illustrates levels too high and too low to allow proper evaluation of treatment effects. For example, in Figure 20a, an increase in percentage of correct /r/ productions to 10% as a function of /r/ training would be difficult to support because correct /r/ productions were

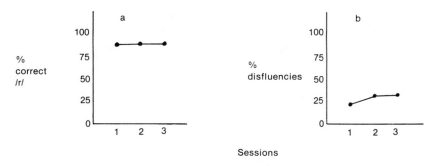

Figure 20. Inappropriate hypothetical baselines for two behaviors. In *a* correct /r/ production is at a high level prior to training of correct /r/, and in *b* disfluency is at a low level before treatment to decrease frequency of occurrence.

already occurring at a high level in baseline. Likewise, a sufficient decrease in percentage of disfluencies to demonstrate treatment effects could not occur because of the low percentage of occurrence already in baseline. The difference between baseline and treatment in both cases would be too small to draw conclusions concerning the effectiveness of training.

No standards have been suggested regarding how high or low rates should be in baseline; that depends largely on the behaviors studied. However, the best criterion an experimenter can apply to determine if the level is appropriate to the question posed is to remember that the data in the B phase must be defended.

Effects Across Phases

Baseline data, of course, are not the only data involved in evaluating treatment effects. Indeed, this can only be done by comparing data from the B phase with data from the A phase.

Similar to the A phase, data are inspected in terms of trend, slope, and level in the B phase. Although data in treatment are examined for these three aspects individually for the B phase, the ultimate decision regarding effects is based on comparisons between A and B phases. It is for this reason that stability in baseline is important. Data in baseline are used to predict performance in the B phase. The prediction is that if the independent variable is not introduced, performance would remain at the baseline level in regard to trend, slope, and level. A change in performance when treatment is introduced therefore provides evidence that the change may be due to treatment. In an A-B-A-B design, performance in the B phase in turn is used to predict performance in the next A phase when the independent variable is no longer present. If performance shifts according to prediction when the independent variable is presented and withdrawn across phases, the experimenter has strong evidence that behavioral change is a function of treatment. Changes across phases, however, must be obvious alterations in terms of trend, slope, and level in performance.

Inasmuch as no set criteria have been proposed, evaluation of treatment effects is sometimes a problem for investigators. Generally, in examining data from within-subject experimental designs, changes across phases must be large enough to allow no room for ambiguous interpretation during visual inspection. As Parsonson and Baer (1978) explain, if effects are so weak that they cannot be readily observed, or need to be teased out by aid of statistics, they are probably equally weak clinically and therefore not useful for adoption as intervention strategies or procedures.

The last point brings up another criterion to be used in evaluating strength of treatment effects, that is, clinical or therapeutic relevance of treatment. As has been pointed out by Kazdin (1977c), a reduction of self-injurious behavior in a psychotic child from 80% to 40% is not clinically significant. In order to be significant therapeutically, reduction would have to be near to a 0% level, because only at this level would a child be behaving normally. By the same token, a similar principle applies in examining data in communicative disorders. Is a reduction in disfluency from 50% to 25% of applied significance, or is an increase in use of pronouns from 5% to 30% an important therapeutic effect?

In the absence of set criteria for evaluating whether experimental control and clinically significant results have been obtained in a study, results of surveys by DeProspero and Cohen (1979) can be offered as guidelines to be used by investigators. Partially, the purpose was to determine criteria used by judges in evaluating studies, and whether agreement in visual judgment could be attributed to any particular aspects of the data.

To explore judgmental interpretation of results, a set of simulated A-B-A-B design graphs were drawn in which various values of three factors commonly used in evaluating single-subject data were depicted. The three values included: 1) patterns of shifts from one phase to the next, 2) degree (amount) of change from one phase to the next, and 3) the trend and slope of the trend in the data. A total of 108 members of the Board of Editors for the *Journal of Applied Behavior Analysis* and *Journal of the Experimental Analysis of Behavior* served as judges in interpreting the graphed data. The surveyors learned that agreement regarding specific criteria used among judges was not high, but that most judges used all three factors in combination rather than a single factor in arriving at a decision concerning treatment effects. A questionnaire about factors used by judges in reaching decisions elicited a number of replies. Most frequently mentioned were "trends" and "slopes" and how they related to the hypothesis under investigation. Trends and slopes were examined both within and between conditions. Levels were also attended to, particularly regarding overlap in levels across phases. Finally, notions of stability and variability within and across conditions were used by some judges.

Thus, no well defined standards for evaluating experimental control or treatment effects are available at present. Furthermore, although similar factors play a part in all judges' decisions, weight given to each differs among individuals. Add to this factors aside from the data, such as number of replications and social significance, and the task becomes more complicated. It is partly this variability in evaluation criteria that has led individuals to suggest statistical aids for evaluating effects when visual inspection is uncertain (DeProspero and Cohen, 1979, Kazdin, 1976; Jones et al., 1978).

Before proceeding to the next topic, we should study some examples of published studies in communicative disorders. The purpose is to illustrate, with a few adequate and less adequate graphs, changes within and across phases in the dependent variable and to discuss the results with regard to evaluative criteria. Not all possible data combinations are presented, primarily because the number of studies is somewhat limited, and because the number of combinations is too large to include in one chapter.

In the following discussion figures are presented with data from published studies in order to examine trends, slopes, and levels. Comments on adequacy of the data according to the three factors, or problems encountered in interpreting the data are included to demonstrate the evaluation process in data examination by visual inspection alone.

The first two examples illustrate adequate baseline and treatment data from an A-B-A-B and multiple-baseline design study. The A-B-A-B study was conducted by Costello and Hurst (1981), who investigated the effect of time-out and a burst of noise on disfluencies. The experimenters were interested in generality, that is, whether punishing one aspect of stuttering behavior would reduce frequency of occurrence of other aspects. Because in our present discussion emphasis is on evaluation of trend, slope, and level of data points within baseline, treatment and reversal phases, and across phases, the entire methodology and study results are not reported. Only data patterns are reproduced and explained. Moreover, three subjects participated in the study but results for just one of the subjects are deemed sufficient for demonstration purposes in this chapter. Therefore, only data for subject 1 are reproduced in Figure 21. Also, for purposes of the present discussion, the C phase is ignored. Tremor disfluencies were consequated for this subject, but both tremors and repetitions measured.

The trend in baseline shows slight variability, but because treatment was directed toward reducing the frequency of the behavior, the slight increase in

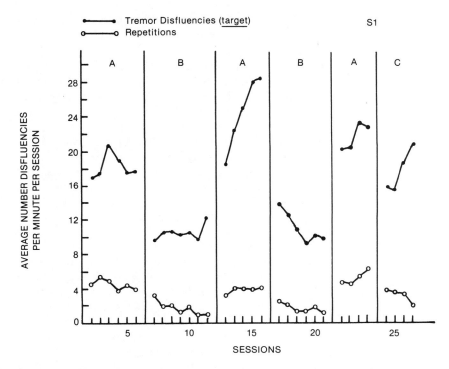

Figure 21. Disfluency data for subject 1. The last data point in each condition is from the same session as the first data point in the subsequent session. Experimental conditions are indicated at the top of the graph and are separated by dark vertical lines. Stuttering topographies measured for subject 1 are defined in the legend. (From Costello and Hurst, 1981, p. 251. Copyright by American Speech-Language-Hearing Association. Reproduced by permission).

the last two data points is in the right direction. The level in baseline is also appropriate in that the behavior has room to move up or down, depending on the effect of the treatment in the B phase.

The dramatic shift in level in the first treatment phase provides the first piece of evidence that the treatment may have effected a change in frequency of disfluencies. Although a slight increase was beginning to appear just before the second A phase, the stability of the decrease in the first treatment phase suggests that treatment continued to be effective.

Naturally, the dramatic shifts in level, slope, and trend in the second A and B phases leave no doubt that treatment was effective. In all phases, the changes in levels provide the strongest evidence for independent variable control. Nevertheless, the appropriate trends and slopes in each of the remaining phases help to support the conclusion that the treatment was responsible for the changes in disfluencies each time. Visual inspection of the data clearly allows interpretation of treatment effectiveness in each A-B-A segment. That the effectiveness was demonstrated across several phases adds elegance and confirms the results.

An excellent example of mutliple-baseline study with clear graphic data was completed by Frisch and Schumaker (1974). The study was concerned with training generalized receptive prepositions. Three prepositional phrases constituted the multiple-baseline design. The dependent variable was generalization to untrained probe items within the prepositional category be-ing trained. Training procedures constituted the independent variable. A graph of the child's performance in the study is reproduced in Figure 22. The child, whose condition was diagnosed as "psychogenic retardation associated with emotional disturbance," was trained to follow instructions containing prepositional phrases, for example, "Put the shovel next to the bucket." After baseline on the three prepositional phrases had been completed, train-ing was introduced on the first phrase, "next to." During training on this phrase, sentences containing the prepositions "under" and "on top of" con-tinued to be tested. When criterion on the first prepositional category was reached, training on the second prepositional category was initiated. When criterion on the second preposition was reached, training shifted to the third prepositional category. The data in the graph are responses to the untrained probe items, that is, generalization data.

Plainly, baseline data show stability with no trend or slope. The level is undoubtedly acceptable. In other words, the child made no correct responses to any of the prepositional instructions. Baseline might be described as perfect for the purpose of the study. With the exception of one correct response to the "on top of" preposition, during "under" training the multi-ple baseline held, as it is supposed to if the behaviors are independent of one another. Obviously, too, the level, trend, and slope in data points changed as training was introduced first on "next to" then on "under" and finally on "on top of." Variability in correct responses to probe items is evident; nonetheless, it is apparent that correct responses were generally at a high level in the category undergoing training. The training procedure, as can be seen in the graph, included progressive steps. First, the "next to" preposition was trained, then "next to" and "under" were alternated before "under" was trained alone. "On top of" was trained alone in the fourth phase and in the final phase the three prepositions were trained simultaneously. Recall that the data displayed in the graph are generalization, not training data, which could account for some of the variability. However, in comparing the trend, slope, and level of the data in the different treatment phases with the pattern of the baseline data it is not difficult to conclude that experimental control was demonstrated across three behaviors and that the training had an effect on generalization.

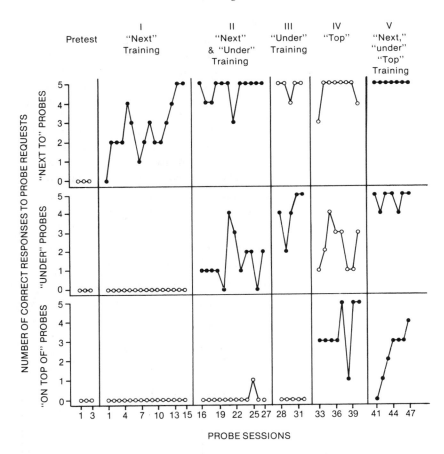

Figure 22. The number of correct responses Johnny made to untrained requests in probe sessions. *Dots* indicate the categories trained within a given condition and *open circles* indicate the categories that were not trained in each condition. (From Frisch and Schumaker, 1974, p. 615. Copyright by Society for the Experimental Analysis of Behavior, Inc. Reproduced by permission).

An example of data in a forced reversal design is found in a study by Johnson and Kaye (1976). A deaf multihandicapped child was trained to speech-read the names of six fruits using tokens, smiles, and signing of "good boy." In the third phase, forced reversal, contingencies were reversed. Now, instead of presenting tokens and praise for correct responses, incorrect responses were praised. In the fourth phase, reinforcement of correct responses was reinstituted. Another treatment was added in the fifth and sixth phases of the study. Because these were not controlled evaluations, data for these phases are not presented, only the first four phases. A portion of the entire graph is presented in Figure 23. The baseline data pattern is less clear in this study than in the first example of a reversal. More than 50% of the responses in the first baseline session are correct, a rather high percentage. The trend across baseline sessions, however, shows a rather sharp downward slope and levels off at approximately 30% correct. The last two data points in baseline are several percentage points above the level obtained in the third session. They evidence a stable pattern; however, the minimum three stable data points would have provided more conclusive evidence that number of correct responses probably would not vary greatly if training were not initiated. Variability in baseline appears to exceed 10% from session 1 to ses-

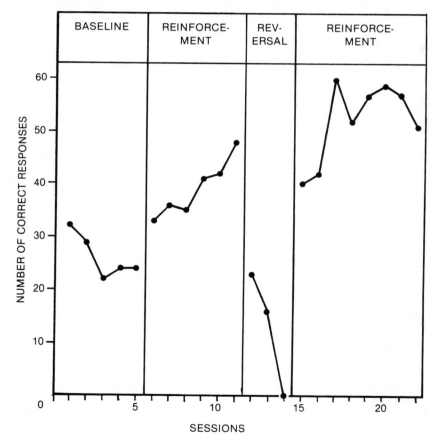

Figure 23. Number of correct responses out of 60 presentations during each of the seven steps of experiment I starting with baseline. (From Johnson and Kaye, 1976, p. 228. Copyright by American Speech-Language-Hearing Association. Reproduced by permission).

sion 3, again, a variation slightly in excess of a comfort level. The slope of the trend in increase of correct responses in treatment is great enough to place more confidence in treatment effects. And of course, the rapid and extreme drop off in correct responses in the reversal phase makes the change in the data pattern even more apparent. The fourth phase data show such a high level of correct responses, and such a large change in level that there is little doubt about treatment effects.

Data are not always as clear as in the previous examples. A linear decrease in frequency across phases is illustrated in a study by Engel and Groth (1976). Six children with articulation errors participated in this study of the effect on sound production of a child monitoring the correctness of his own response. Actually, the study consisted of two treatments administered sequentially in the same order, not counterbalanced across subjects. Of interest to the present discussion is the data pattern displayed in the graph in Figure 24. Baseline consisted of seven sessions, a more than adequate sample. In each session, the child's misarticulations were counted as he or she read during a classroom reading period. When baseline measures had been completed, the child was administered treatment. The first treatment consisted of reinforcing the child's correct productions during reading in the clinic. Each session lasted 20 minutes; however, the first 5 minutes of reading formed the data base. These counts were labeled *overt* counts. Additionally, the observer continued to count misarticulations in the classroom reading periods and these counts were called *covert* counts. Incorrect productions during the first 5 minutes were counted; treatment continued for an additional 15 minutes but data on performance were not collected. The treatment lasted for 10 sessions. The second treatment was introduced in the eleventh session. In this treatment phase the child continued to read, but each time a word with the target sound was produced the child was asked to raise his or her hand if the target sound was produced correctly. Correct judgments and productions were followed by reinforcement, presumably the same reinforcement administered in the first treatment phase, although the investigators do not state this. The data presented in the graphs consisted of percentage of incorrect productions during the first 5 minutes of each session. The second treatment continued until the percentage of misarticulations reached 5% or lower for five consecutive sessions. A follow-up measurement was included in the study. In this phase, which lasted 10 sessions, the child's incorrect productions during classroom reading were counted. The follow-up measurement condition was similar to the baserate condition; that is, incorrect productions in the classroom were counted but not treated. Results for one child are reproduced from the study in Figure 24. Although individual graphs for the six children were included in the article in which the study is reported, only one graph is reproduced here because the other five graphs are similar to this one.

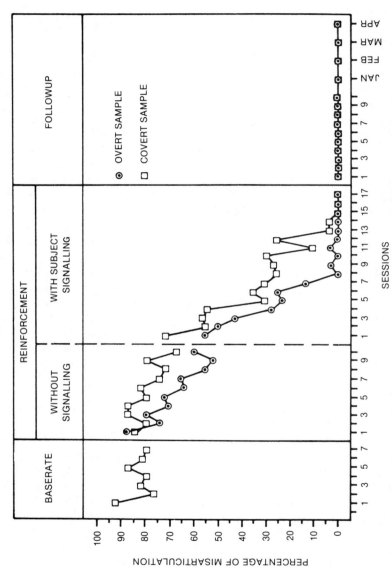

Figure 24. Percentage of misarticulation before, during, and after reinforcement of correct articulatory production, first without and then with subject signaling: subject 5. (From Engel and Groth, 1976, p. 98. Copyright by American Speech-Language-Hearing Association. Reproduced by permission).

The baserate data will be examined first. Recall that the treatment was to result in a decrease in the percentage of incorrect productions. Without a doubt, the child was producing errors at a high rate in baserate, so level was certainly adequate. Neither was variability a problem; most of the data points are within a 10% variation range. The trend is somewhat ambiguous for the purpose of the study in that the last two data points show a decreasing trend. It is possible to ask whether the decrease would have continued if baseline measurement had continued and no treatment was introduced. Additional baseline measurements might have dispelled the ambiguity if they showed that the decrease ceased. When treatment was initiated in the B phase, the decreasing trend showed a moderate slope with slight variability, suggesting that treatment may have functioned to decrease incorrect responding. When the second treatment was introduced the trend continued at a sharper slope. The sharp decrease could again be interpreted as support for the effectiveness of the treatment. This interpretation is open to question in viewing the data from the follow-up measure in which treatment was withdrawn. A shift in level, slope, and trend in an opposite direction from the treatment phase is not evident. Indeed, the linear decrease continued and remained at zero level. A complete elimination of incorrect responses is certainly a clinical triumph. But the variable or variables responsible for the elimination are not readily identified. In order to demonstrate experimental control, that is, treatment effects, data must show changes from one phase to the next as conditions alternate. This is not to say treatment was ineffective, only that treatment effects were not isolated according to the data presented. Essentially, the study becomes an A-B design in which the effect of the intervention may be conjectured but is not supported with evidence. The linearly decreasing trend and slope in error percentage from baseline to follow-up makes it difficult to separate treatment effects from other variables operating during the course of the study, such as passage of time and events at home or in the classroom. Results of the study are encouraging, however, and could lead to designing a controlled evaluation to demonstrate that treatment was indeed responsible for eliminating error responses.

In the *Journal of Communication Disorders,* a study by Costello and Ferrer (1976) of several treatments administered sequentially offered complicated data for inspection. Six children participated; detailed data were presented for two and data for one of the two subjects is reproduced in Figure 25.

In short, the study was designed to explore if "punishment" functioned to reduce articulation errors during articulation training. Correct responses in training were followed by tokens presented by the experimenter. A predetermined number of tokens enabled the child to purchase a toy.

Three procedures for incorrect responses served as independent variables. Briefly, they were 1) the experimenter saying "No" in a mod-

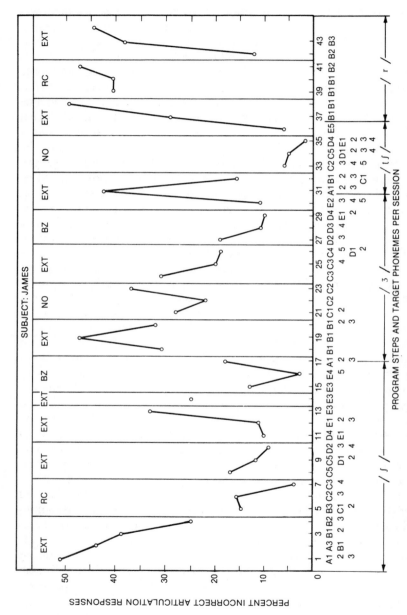

Figure 25. The effects of all experimental conditions on the percent of incorrect articulation responses for James. (From Costello and Ferrer, 1976, p. 52. Copyright by American Elsevier Publishing Company, Inc. Reproduced by permission).

erately loud tone, 2) a 1-second buzzer sound, and 3) withdrawal of a token. These treatments for incorrect responses were alternated with a "no-punishment" condition in which incorrect responses were ignored. This condition, according to the authors, simulated an extinction phase, that is, a return to baseline conditions. Each phase was in effect for three sessions regardless of the response pattern within a condition. One exception to this format was institution of a second extinction condition in case a subject's incorrect responses remained too low. In this condition both correct and incorrect responses were ignored. (More information on designs for exploring two or more treatments in one study can be found in Chapter 6.)

As labeled on the ordinate in Figure 25, the dependent variable was percent incorrect productions. The proposed "punishment" procedures were evaluated for effectiveness in decreasing incorrect articulation responses during training. The phases are labeled on the graph and include: Ext, extinction; RC, response cost—loss of a token; Bz, 1-second buzzer; and No, experimenter saying "No" in a moderately loud tone. Each "punishment" phase is preceded and followed by at least one extinction phase.

The data in the phases will not be analyzed comprehensively; neither will the phases be examined individually. Rather, the intent is to draw attention to a few patterns that can be used in reaching decisions about what the data show.

The first is the sharply decreasing trend in the data for the first extinction phase. Before "punishment" was introduced, incorrect responses had decreased from approximately a 52% to a 25% level. Treatment was introduced when incorrect responses were occurring at a low and decreasing rate. A similar pattern can be observed within and across other phases of the experiment.

Variability occurs within and across phases. Likely, the investigators designed equal phases in keeping with the suggestion by Hersen and Barlow (1976) to minimize confounding from unequal phases. Practical considerations must also have entered into the decision because the entire experiment required a large number of phases. Perhaps, in order to conserve time, the experiment was kept within a reasonable time limit and length of phases was set at three sessions. The variability in percentage of incorrect responses that occurred may have been unexpected, so that problems in interpreting the data could not be foreseen. Once observed, it might have been possible to implement the flexibility inherent in within-subject designs by changing to a stability criterion for terminating each phase.

A pattern mentioned briefly but not illustrated in the studies discussed previously is overlap of data points across phases. A few instances of overlap are found in Figure 25. For example, overlap occurs between the response cost phase in condition 2 and extinction in phase 3, and in the "No" condition and extinction condition in phases 8 and 9. Overlap of data across phases suggests equal effects in each phase irrespective of presence or absence of the independent variable. Generally speaking, at times one or more punishment conditions appear to reveal a greater reduction in error responses than the extinction conditions; however, the data are elusive. To the credit of the investigators, several of the problems are recognized in the discussion and qualifications regarding treatment effectiveness are offered.

Implications

Hopefully, the five examples of data patterns from published studies offer guidelines for evaluating data in single-subject experimental studies. The examples should also show why there is discussion about the form of data analysis to be used when data are difficult to interpret. The viewpoint set forth in this book is that visual inspection of raw data conforms most closely to the rationale of within-subject research. To conclude that experimental control has been demonstrated and treatment effects are apparent, data patterns, clearly, should reveal appropriate changes across conditions with a sufficient number of data points to establish stability of the behavior. If evaluation is difficult or uncertain, it may be best to conclude that the treatment may not be effective. This is a conservative view and the criteria are stringent. But perhaps, as Parsonson and Baer (1978) have noted, the conservative view should reveal only strong variables that in the end will be the variables contributing to development of successful intervention programs.

EVALUATION CRITERIA ACROSS STUDIES

In within-subject research, as in all experimental studies, generality of findings is an important issue. A criticism frequently leveled at single-subject studies is that generality of findings is limited due to the number of subjects studied, that is, $N = 1$. Investigators operating within the rationale of group studies and statistical designs object to generalizing treatment effectiveness to a group of clients from results of a single client. Obviously, one subject is not representative of all individuals suffering from a particular disorder. Within-subject researchers have not quarrelled with this premise, and their answer to these criticisms comes in the form of replications. Broadly defined, replication refers to reproduction of the experiment or repetition of the experimental procedure. Hersen and Barlow (1976) and others (Michael, 1974a, b; Johnston and Pennypacker, 1980) make a case for superiority of replications over group designs and statistical treatment of data for providing evidence of generality, but the controversy continues. The following pages are devoted to a discussion of replication in within-subject designs, not a review of the controversial issues. Replications are necessary to evaluation of treatment effectiveness.

Replication comes in different forms generally placed under two categories: direct and systematic replication (Sidman, 1960). Hersen and Barlow (1976) have added a third category labeled *clinical replication*. The first two categories of replication are described in this section and examples from communicative research literature are included when available and appropriate. Clinical replication is reserved for discussion within the third category concerning clinical and social significance.

Direct Replication

Sidman divides direct replication into two classes: repetition of the same experiment on one subject and repetition of an experiment on more than one subject. Hersen and Barlow (1976) have defined direct replication: "Direct replication in applied research refers to administration of a given treatment by the same investigator or group of investigators in a specific setting...on a series of clients homogeneous for a particular behavior disorder..." (p. 318).

Direct replication is tied closely to reliability of the treatment procedure; that is, the treatment shown to be effective more often is more certainly a reliable procedure (Hersen and Barlow, 1976). Moreover, direct replication is relevant to establishing generality of a treatment to individuals with similar problems to the subject in the experiment. Hersen and Barlow (1976) caution, however, that generality from direct replication is restricted to statements concerning the population studied. Generalizations about the effectiveness of the treatment when administered by other experimenters or in other settings are not possible from direct replications.

A point to keep in mind is that all within-subject designs have built into them one or another form of replication. The first kind of direct replication proposed by Sidman (repetition of the same experiment on one subject) forms an integral component in an A-B-A-B design. In this design the second A-B replicates the first A-B pair. True, the components are designed to provide experimental control for evaluating effectiveness of treatment, not to demonstrate generality. Nevertheless, an A-B-A-B study conforms to one of Sidman's definitions of direct replication. Primarily, repetition of the baseline and treatment in an A-B-A-B design adds reliable evidence that the treatment is effective if results from the second administration parallel those from the first. Generality information from an A-B-A-B study is limited; namely, that the treatment is not restricted to one successful administration on one subject. It is evidence of treatment effectiveness.

Direct replication across other subjects occurs outside the internal components of a design and is the most frequent form of replication in within-subject research. It is not unusual to find studies involving four subjects: an original and three replications. Even though at times more subjects may be included, four is common. Indeed, it has been recommended that three replications (a total of four subjects) are adequate and additional replications would result in diminishing returns (Hersen and Barlow, 1976). Not that additional data are unwelcome, but they do not necessarily strengthen statements regarding generality of findings to other individuals with similar disorders. If three successful replications are obtained, generality to similar clients is accepted with greater confidence, and effectiveness of the treatment has been demonstrated.

What is involved in a direct replication across subjects? Hersen and Barlow specify that the subjects must be homogeneous, the experimenter the same, and the setting unchanged in conducting a direct replication. We examine the first criterion, homogeneous subjects, in some detail in relation to communicative disorders research. The other two criteria are self-evident and should cause few problems.

In communicative disorders studies, meeting the first criterion is not always easy. Matching clients on relevant variables may prove difficult because of variation in individuals exhibiting the same speech or hearing disorder. Frankly, it is an impossible task to match subjects on all variables. To comply as closely as possible with this requirement, however, an investigator examines all variables carefully with a view toward selecting subject characteristics for matching. The decision entails choosing possible confounding variables and matching subjects on those, while relinquishing a match on variables of less importance. Accurate choices by the investigator are important. For example, an obvious matching variable in language training studies of language-impaired clients is hearing. Normal hearing has to be established for all subjects in case one subject performs differently from the others. If subjects have been matched on hearing, the investigator can determine that performance is not confounded by a subject with a hearing loss. Unfortunately, all matching variables are not as readily identified as hearing. Investigators give serious thought to physical, mental, and social factors, and to the importance of background and history in seeking variables to be controlled, that is, to be matched. Naturally, the behavior to be studied influences selection of matching variables. Therefore, familiarity with a disorder is crucial to the experimenter for designing a well controlled study free from confounding due to subject characteristics.

Admittedly, obtaining homogeneous subjects for direct replication is not always possible. Recognizing that all variables may not be taken into account in developing a study, the experimenter nevertheless matches wherever possible. Problems in matching may be compensated partially by obtaining an exhaustive measure during baseline of the behavior to be treated. By exhaustive, we mean a baseline providing a clear and complete description of the behavior, achieving performance stability within a narrow range of variation, and extending baseline over a reasonable period of time. If subjects are matched closely on baseline performance, the investigator can at least feel comfortable that all performed similarly on the behavior of interest before training even if they differed on other characteristics.

An experimenter need not despair if matching subjects creates problems. Two avenues are open even when subjects differ from each other. The first is a relatively frequently used alternative. It is to conduct the study with the subjects noting differences among them. Surely risk is attached to this alternative, but investigators often have reason to believe that their treatment is powerful enough to override influences from subject characteristics. Indeed, if the assumption proves true and success is achieved with all subjects, regardless of differences, the investigator's faith is rewarded by evidence of generality broader than would have been obtained if subjects had been matched closely. Results would indicate that the treatment is not limited to a small, homogeneous group of clients, but applies to a larger, diverse group. Undeniably, the risk that all subjects will not be affected similarly by the treatment is real. If that occurs, cause for the failure would be unclear. Was it the treatment procedure, or some characteristic inherent in the subjects who were unchanged by treatment?

Herein lies an opportunity to put into execution the second alternative. Following Sidman's (1960) suggestion, the investigator may begin a search for the source(s) of variability. Exploration may begin in examination of characteristics differentiating successful from unsuccessful subjects, or, as some investigators prefer, examination of performance differences starting with baseline and proceeding to performance during training. It is Sidman's (1960) premise that a successful analysis of human behavior will be achieved only after carefully pursuing causes for intersubject variability. Incidentally, behavior analysts who defend visual graphing of data, eschewing use of statistics, often offer an explanation similar to Sidman's. They contend that individual variability should not be ignored when present. On the contrary, effort should be directed at identifying responsible variables and bringing them under experimental control (Parsonson and Baer, 1978; Michael, 1974a and b). This point is emphasized by Johnston and Pennypacker (1980). These authors prefer omitting use of generic terms such as *reversal* or *multiple baseline* in favor of defining basic components that can be combined in an infinite number of arrangements to allow experimenters to change and alter designs when necessary to explore variability. We will never understand human behavior or develop effective intervention programs, they say, if statistics are used to hide intersubject variation. Whether we like it or not, it exists; it will not disappear through statistical manipulation. It may not be visible, but it is there. Flexibility to explore variability among subjects in within-subject designs has been lauded by behavior analysts.

Generality from direct replication allows experimenters to postulate the permissable range of subject variability for treatment success. It does not provide evidence on subject performance in the presence of other experimenters or in other settings. Such evidence requires systematic replication.

Systematic Replication

Systematic replication has been defined by Hersen and Barlow (1976) to involve ''. . . exploring the effects of different settings, therapists or clients on a procedure previously demonstrated as successful in a direct replication series'' (p. 62). More precisely, systematic replication consists of varying situations, behavior change agents, clients, or disorders, either singly or in combination, to determine if treatment continues to be effective when these variables are changed.

Recollect that direct replications are intended for exploration of generality to other clients with the same disorder, and should be completed before systematic replications are undertaken. Recall also that direct replications give limited information regarding generality of treatment. Systematic replications are required if broader evidence of generality is sought. Therefore, systematic replications are important to establishing overall effectiveness of a treatment.

The importance of systematic replication may have been overlooked in research in behavior disorders. Certainly it is virtually unknown in communicative disorders research. Yet, it happens in an unplanned manner in some instances, as when an investigator designs a number of studies to explore more than one facet of a single question. Or, it occurs when the investigator, in order to fulfull requirements of a study design, is forced to send more than one assistant to administer treatment to subjects in different settings, for example, a rehabilitation clinic, a school, and a hospital. The result is that, although the investigator may be primarily interested in direct replication, circumstances force systematic replication to occur simultaneously. An example of a series of studies not specifically designed as systematic replications, but which might meet criteria for both direct and systematic replication, is presented at the end of this section.

Whereas in direct replication comparison is between treatment and no treatment with homogeneous subjects, systematic replication compares the effect of one treatment across other behaviors, settings, clients, and clinicians. In other words, in a direct replication variables other than treatment are held constant, whereas in systematic replication other variables are changed.

It should be noted that different clients are involved in both direct and systematic replications. The difference is that clients are matched closely in direct replications, but in systematic replications heterogeneity is allowed and sometimes encouraged. Therefore, amount of variation helps to define whether replication is direct or systematic. Classification of a replication into one or the other category is not always easy. For instance, variation between clients is on a continuum. An investigator may select clients differing from each other on only one or two characteristics, on several characteristics, or totally. To what degree should clients differ from each other to classify the study a systematic replication? No guidelines have been proposed, and the question might be a moot one; heretogeneity is more common than homogeneity in clients with the same disorder, even when direct replications are sought. It is difficult to find clients differing from each other on only one or two characteristics. The point is that systematic replication may be more common than heretofore thought. If so, perhaps we could make stronger statements concerning generality than we previously thought possible. An investigator would be well advised to examine subject characteristics carefully in initiating direct replications; the differences between subjects might be large enough to qualify the replication as systematic with broader generality to treatment of the disorder than if it were classified as a direct replication.

A similar point can be made regarding replications across behaviors. Communicative disorders, as well as clients exhibiting them, vary along a continuum. At one end of the continuum, subjects with the same disorder differing topographically on only one or two dimensions may be selected, or they may differ on several dimensions. At the other end of the continuum an investigator may choose subjects with totally different disorders. We might ask again how greatly behaviors have to differ in order to classify a replication as systematic. Perhaps a number of replications considered to be direct could actually qualify as systematic because of differences in behaviors treated. A possibility to be considered is that generality across behaviors occurs more frequently than hitherto credited in single-subject studies of communicative disorders.

An element of systematic replication is present whenever a multiple baseline design is used if the criteria set forth by Hersen and Barlow (1976) are applied. As previously explained, a multiple-baseline study may be designed across behaviors, across subjects, or across settings, aspects also varied in systematic replications. The only variable that can be varied in systematic replication but not in mutiple-baseline designs is experimenters. Behavior change agents have not been used to form the control in multiple-baseline designs. Nevertheless, we may view most multiple-baseline designs as a beginning in systematic replication.

Contrary to direct replications, no limit has been set on the number of systematic replications needed to demonstrate generality across settings, clients, clinicians, and behaviors. Indeed, systematic replications can continue for years because of the number and combinations of variables that can be manipulated. Not only are settings and clinicians varied, so is the amount by which clients and behaviors differ from one replication to another. All these replications take time, and investigators seldom wait for the conclusion of systematic replications before applying the treatment in therapeutic circumstances.

Before moving to a discussion of the third category of evaluation criteria, criteria for concluding that replications support generality must be discussed. A brief section addresses the issue of interpretation of replication results.

Replications are used to predict treatment effectiveness to clients, settings, disorders, and clinicians, that is, generality. In group studies random sampling and factorial designs are used for this purpose. In within-subject research the number of replications needed to support generality of treatment has not been specified for systematic replications. Hersen and Barlow's (1976) proposal of three direct replications is based on their experience as researchers not on quantifiable data from direct study of generality. If treatment effects are strong and uniform when a study has been conducted with four subjects, Hersen and Barlow (1976) observed that additional data added little new information concerning generality to other clients in behavior disorders research. Three successful replications (a total of four subjects) provide the investigator with sufficient data to predict success with similar subjects.

It is another matter when mixed results are obtained, two options are available to the investigator. One, differences between the successfully and unsuccessfully treated subjects are examined in the hope of identifying variables responsible for the different results. Flexibility of within-subject designs allows the experimenter to alter the study design immediately if a probable variable is located. When the alteration is completed, subjects failing to benefit from the original treatment are administered the modified procedure. If the changed treatment is successful, replications with homogeneous subjects can begin. Another option is examination of differences; and, if the responsible variable appears to be a subject characteristic, clients more homogeneous to the original subject can be sought. Treatment can then be administered to the new subjects for replication purposes. Later, the investigator may return to the unsuccessful subjects to explore alternative procedures.

Aside from Hersen and Barlow's (1976) suggestion, no specific criteria have been advanced for predicting generality across clients, disorders, clinicians, and settings. This may be partly due to the lack of empirical data on replications, particularly systematic replications. Single-subject research does not have a long and abundant history, so it may take time for data to accumulate and patterns to emerge allowing for greater specificity regarding requirements for statements of generality and effectiveness of treatment over a broad range of subjects and situations.

At present, investigators use information available to them from within-subject studies, drawing from their own experiences as researchers to reach decisions. Comfort level differs among experimenters; some require no more than one replication if strong effects are found, whereas others demand several uniform replications. For now, perhaps the largest contribution within-subject researchers can make is to provide comprehensive descriptions of subjects, procedures, and results, whether successes or failures. The information would aid other researchers in designing original treatment studies, but more importantly, in deciding the form and number of replications needed to infer generality.

A series of studies on coarticulatory or contextual effects in articulation training constitutes an example of direct and systematic replication in research in communicative disorders. The studies were completed by several investigators (Elbert and McReynolds, 1975, 1978; Rigor, 1980; and McReynolds, 1980).

Before describing the studies a brief background and rationale are offered. From descriptive studies of children with articulation errors it was discovered that children sometimes produce the error sound correctly. Analysis of their correct and incorrect productions revealed that the error sound was correctly produced in the context of particular surrounding sounds, that is, in particular phonetic contexts. The /s/, for instance, was produced correctly more often when followed by another consonant than by a vowel. Further, preceding sounds appeared to have no influence on how the error sound was produced, but following sounds did. Moreover, the /s/ and /z/ were produced correctly more often when they were followed by a plosive sound (e.g., /p/, /b/, /t/, /d/, /k/, and /g/) than when they were followed by a fricative or affricate sound (e.g., /s/, /z/, /f/, /v/, /tʃ/, etc.). Contextual influences were also identified for /r/ production in children who misarticulated /r/.

Results from these descriptive studies led investigators to suggest that certain phonetic contexts were universally facilitative for learning to produce /s/, /z/, or /r/, and certain contexts were neutral or even inhibitory to efficient acquisition of the sounds. Clinicians were encouraged to take advantage of the facilitative contexts in training children with articulation disorders. The implication, of course, is that a child acquires a target sound more rapidly and efficiently if the facilitative sounds are used in training items.

The value of these contexts in treatment was explored in the coarticulatory training studies to be reported. To do this, a number of within-subject design studies were conducted. The dependent variable in all studies was correct articulation of the target sound in untrained syllables, words, and phrases composed of the proposed facilitative, neutral or inhibiting contexts (sounds). The target sound was embedded in the contexts. The untrained items were presented during /r/, /s/, or /z/ training to children who had produced these sounds incorrectly before training. Generalization of correct production of the target sound to the untrained contexts was tested frequently to obtain data on patterns of target sound acquisition in the generalization items as training progressed.

In the first study a multiple-baseline design across groups was used (Elbert and McReynolds, 1975). All children misarticulated the /r/ sound. Six children received training, while the remaining six served as controls. When the first six had completed training the second six were started in training. The /r/ was trained in four different contexts in nonsense syllables. Each child was trained on only one context, but each training context was replicated across at least one other child. The contexts were assigned randomly within each group. Generalization was tested to all four contexts. Training procedures consisted of imitation in which reinforcement was shifted from a continuous to a variable ratio schedule. The untrained contexts were probed during training but responses to these contexts were not reinforced. Results showed that the children generalized to all contexts tested. No particular context evoked more correct responses than another.

The next study was designed to explore generalization of the /s/ sound (Elbert and McReynolds, 1978). An A-B-A-B design was used and the study consisted of one experiment with four replications, a total of five subjects. A variety of phonetic contexts formed the generalization items providing a greater opportunity for contextual influences to occur. Moreover, in this study both imitative and spontaneous responses were evoked to determine if contextual effects were tied to the manner in which responses were elicited. Several training items were administered to insure stable correct production of the target sound during generalization testing. As in the first study, generalization to untrained items occurred, but contextual influences did not appear. Children displayed generalization patterns unrelated to phonetic contexts; the patterns were individual to each child.

Two additional studies were completed to explore contextual effects: another study on /r/ production (Rigor, 1980) and another on /s/ and /z/ production (McReynolds, 1980). In the /r/ study, the generalization items included a variety of phonetic contexts in which /r/ was tested both within and across words. A limited number of items had been included in the first

/r/ study and only imitation had been tested before. In the study by Rigor (1980), children were given an opportunity to respond to imitated and spontaneous items. Thus, the study was designed to provide more opportunities for contextual effects to appear. An A-B-A-B design with four misarticulating children was used. Training procedures were similar to procedures in the previous studies.

The final /s/ and /z/ study was conducted as a multiple-baseline design across behaviors (phonemes) with counterbalancing of the behaviors (McReynolds 1980). A total of six children received training: three learned first to produce /s/ and three learned to produce /z/ first. Coarticulation influences were tested across words in phrases in which the /s/ or /z/ was preceded and followed by nasal, plosive, fricative, and affricate consonants as well as representative vowels. One hundred twenty generalization items were presented at each testing to each child throughout training.

The final /r/ study and the /s/ and /z/ study replicated results obtained in the first two studies. No phonetic context or contexts stood out as facilitating or inhibiting. Children generalized to all contexts, and although children presented generalization patterns, the patterns differed among them. Universal contexts were not identified. None of the patterns were related to particular contexts in the generalization items.

This series of studies does not conform to the usual pattern in within-subject designs in which training is the independent variable and a change in the behavior directly treated forms the dependent variable. That is, acquisition of the /r/, /s/ or /z/ in the training items was not explored; it was assured. Generalization of the trained sound, if it occurred, would evidence a pattern that could be traced to contexts used in testing generalization, creating an indirect measure of training. Basically, the studies were designed as A-B-A-B or multiple-baseline studies, but another component in the form of a probe was added. The probe tested the behavior of interest but was not a measure of the behavior in the training context. More will be said about designs appropriate for generalization studies in a later chapter, designs especially appealing to communicative disorders researchers.

The contextual studies, although different from common forms of within-subject studies, are reported in this section because they illustrate replication series rather well. Unfortunately, replication series devoted to study of one variable are rare, perhaps nonexistent, in speech-language pathology and audiology.

Direct replication is obvious in the reported studies. Each study included a minimum of one experimental subject and three or more replications. Within each study subjects were matched on measures thought by the investigators to form possible confounding variables. The children were within a narrow age range, and had been diagnosed as children with functional articulation disorders, otherwise functioning normally in school and at home. None of the children had hearing, language, or academic problems; they came from monolingual homes. Moreover, an effort was made to restrict the number of error sounds each child produced in addition to /r/, /s/, and /z/. Stimulability was tested, as was error consistency. Baseline in each study was defined narrowly and measures continued until stability was reached. Therefore, the children in each study were matched as closely as possible on subject characteristics and on articulatory behavior, a criterion for direct replication. The same training procedures were administered to the subjects in each study and, therefore, another criterion for direct replication was met.

Criteria for systematic replication were also met. Replication occurred across investigators and settings in several ways. The studies were conducted by more than one investigator and/or research assistant. Settings included public schools, private schools, and the laboratory. Replication also occurred across behaviors. In two studies generalization of the /r/ sound was explored, in one study /s/ was evaluated, and in the final study both /s/ and /z/ were investigated. Thus, replication occurred across settings, behavior change agents, clients, and behaviors. Replication across disorders was not obtained. A replication across disorders might have involved a subject population with organic problems, such as cleft palate. More appropriately, however, it would involve subjects with a different diagnosis, for instance, language disorders. Nevertheless, sufficient direct and systematic replications were obtained to allow generalization to clients with articulation problems in other circumstances. The conclusion was that coarticulatory effects, if present, are individual to clients and too subtle to be useful for selecting training contexts in articulation treatment. Because universal contexts were not revealed, the series of studies indicated that clinicians could select contexts suitable to individual clients for target sound training.

It appeared that another variable, or variables, had a stronger influence on generalization patterns in clients with articulation problems. The investigators' attention can now turn toward identification of the variable or variables responsible for articulation generalization. As a matter of fact, from the series of studies a number of variables may stand out as potentially relevant. Recall that results evidenced considerable individual variability. It is possible, for example, to trace individual generalization patterns of children, because the data are available. The investigators also have detailed information on the subjects if they wish to pursue subject differences. Furthermore, they have considerable data on each child's responses to the generalization items throughout training if they wish to look for variables related to progress in generalization. Moreover, detailed training data are available if the investigators desire to examine differences in acquisition of the target sounds. The investigators have a wealth of information for launching a search of variables related to articulation generalization. At this point, then, the experimenters can use their experience, their data, and information from articulation literature to select the most plausible variable or variables to study. They have the advantage of examining a comprehensive set of data from a controlled replication series—systematic and systematically obtained data.

CLINICAL AND SOCIAL EVALUATION

It is inherent in applied experimental analysis that treatments found effective in single variable studies be tested in broader, more complex contexts to explore whether behavior changes are maintained in other situations. Without a demonstration that a behavior change is maintained and extended to a client's everyday functioning in other settings, applied researchers should continue to have reservations about treatment effectiveness. Criteria in the third evaluation category are directed toward providing evidence of generality to the subject as a complete person and to environments other than the clinic. Included in the third category are clinical replication and social validation. Each will be discussed individually.

Clinical Replication

Clinical replication consists of "...an advanced replication procedure in which a treatment 'package' containing two or more distinctive procedures is available to a succession of clients with multiple behaviors or emotional problems that cluster together" (Hersen and Barlow, 1976; p. 335). 'Cluster' refers to a diagnostic label including a number of factors, as in "childhood autism."

A clinical replication comes about after extensive research has been completed in exploring treatment variables. When a sufficient number of relevant variables have been identified, they are grouped together into a package containing several procedures. Note the word "cluster." It refers to the multifaceted profile of a diagnostic label. A stutterer, for instance, may exhibit several behavioral manifestations of his stuttering problem and, additionally, display attitudinal, emotional, or personality problems. A treatment package for these stutterers would consist of several treatments aimed at modification of the stuttering as well as other problems. Before the package was compiled, however, each treatment would have been evaluated individually. Obviously, a package or technique evolves gradually over years of controlled studies. It has been suggested that group designs may be more efficacious than within-subject designs for testing treatment packages (Hersen and Barlow, 1976). Initially, single-subject designs are used to study individual treatments; this is called technique building. Later, group designs are used to test the entire package; this is labeled *technique testing*.

Because no treatment packages have been developed in this manner in communicative disorders, an in-depth discussion of clinical replication procedures will not be attempted here. In fact, clinical replication is rare in the behavior disorders literature as a whole. It is desirable, however, to keep in mind the steps by which treatment programs can be developed and evaluated in a controlled manner. Clinicians can place more confidence in programs derived from scientifically obtained data than from opinions based on hunches and clinical intuition.

Social Validation

Behavioral research today is broader in scope than was envisioned fifteen years ago. The move is from exclusively laboratory studies to research in the natural environment. Moreover, researchers are beginning to ask if behavior changes obtained in controlled experiments are observed in social contexts (Kazdin, 1977c; Van Houten, 1979 and Wolf, 1978).

Behavioral researchers have moved to a greater appreciation of the need to demonstrate that behavioral changes carry over into everyday living, and that others can describe these changes. It is a move toward social validation, and social validation may be considered one of the criteria to be met for demonstrating treatment effectiveness. According to Wolf (1978), three questions must be answered in judging social validity: 1) Are the behavioral goals those wanted by society? 2) Do others in the environment concur that the treatment procedures are appropriate and acceptable? and 3) Are the subjects and others in the environment satisfied with the results?

Answers to these questions have been explored on two levels. First is an attempt to take commonly used subjective labels, define them operationally, and measure them objectively. Second is the effort to measure treatment effects in everyday situations by having clients and behaviors rated by others, sometimes in subjective terms. Each level has more than one form or procedure, sometimes overlapping each other. They are illustrated briefly in this section.

Subjective Terms   People tend to describe individuals and interactions in subjective terms, for example, "an affectionate person," "satisfying experience." On the whole, experimental analysts have avoided such terms owing to difficulty in operationally defining and objectively measuring them. But the terms are common and apparently meaningful to subjects and others in describing treatments, behaviors, and clients. Interest in social validation does not allow avoiding contact with the terms; and, therefore, the terms have become the focus of research endeavors. The purpose is to obtain as clear a definition of terms as possible, then develop measuring tools to gather data on treatment effectiveness.

A good example of such research is a study by Braukmann, Kirigin, and Wolf (1976), conducted in the Achievement Place Research Project in which youths are trained to function appropriately in the environment. Training is conducted by teaching-parents. When community members and youths were asked what characteristics were important for effective teaching-parents, the answer was that trainers needed to show "warmth." Asked to define "warmth" further, responders stated it was "someone who knows how to relate to youths." Starting with this definition the experimenters set out to identify behaviors teaching-parents needed in order to "relate to youths." Initially some nonverbal behaviors were identified from studies exploring parameters of "empathy" (Haase and Tepper, 1972). Simultaneously youths examined videotaped examples of teaching-parents/youths interactions. While watching the samples the youths listed things they liked and disliked in the interactions. Their responses were placed into categories and rated by youths from A to F. Behaviors rated as A, highly desirable, such as offers to help, joking, explanations, politeness were then taught to teaching-parent trainees. It was found that youths rated the trainers much higher after the teaching-parents had been instructed on the A-rated behaviors. Thus, the experimenters attempted operationally to define "warmth" and corroborated the definition by subjective evaluations from clients.

Subjective terms are also used when treatment effectiveness outside of the experimental setting is judged by others in the environment. In one form it may consist of using a subjective term describing the client and the client's behavior and rating the degree to which the quality in the term is present. An example of this use of subjective terms is found in a study by Jones and Azrin (1969). The investigators developed an apparatus set to a rhythmic beat for the purpose of controlling stuttering. In laboratory studies stutterers were trained to match their speech rate to the beat of a metronome. By doing so, disfluency was controlled and speech rate modified. The apparatus was altered to allow disfluent speakers to wear it to control stuttering during everyday activities. The apparatus worked in the normal environmental situation except that listeners complained the speech sounded artificial. To solve this problem Jones and Azrin made samples of stutterer's speech matched across a variety of beat durations. The various duration samples were submitted to a panel of judges requested to rate the "naturalness" of the speech at each duration. After learning the beat at which speech sounded most natural, the investigators adopted that beat for use in the apparatus. Thus, effectiveness of treatment was socially validated when the apparatus worked outside the experimental setting, and social importance further increased when the speech was modified to sound more pleasing to others.

Extension to Normalcy Therapeutic criterion is used to determine whether behavior changes are appropriate and extensive enough to satisfy the client and society (Kazdin, 1977c). It is directed toward inquiring whether improvement is adequate to everyday functioning as evaluated by the subject and others interacting with the subject. The issue, of course, is the clinical and social importance of a behavioral change. The more direct question is whether the change achieved in treatment is sufficient to enable both the individual involved and the community to perceive the behavior to be occurring within the normal range. The question is appropriate, but "normal range" is not readily defined. Two methods for measuring clinical and social importance have been proposed (Kazdin, 1977c and Van Houten, 1979); social comparison and subjective evaluation. Several procedures may be used in both methods. Two procedures for subjective evaluation are presented in the previous section.

In social comparison the behavior of the individual before and after treatment is compared with the behavior of nondeviant peers who did not need treatment. If the subject's performance falls within a normal range, the treatment is considered successful. For social comparison individuals judged competent in the behavior are selected and their performance level determined (Van Houten, 1979). Instead of average performance, however, best performance is obtained from a selected group in order to provide the optimal level as a standard for treatment success.

Establishing normative targets requires a series of procedures. Initially, competent individuals may be found by asking others frequently in contact with the behavior of interest, such as teachers, parents, employers, and clinicians, to identify competent persons. Measures must be selected to assess presence of variables named, and it is essential that appropriate measures are used for evaluating the behavior and performance level. Corroboration of relevant variables identified by observers may then be obtained through experimental evaluation. It is possible, for example, to manipulate the behavior of interest over a wide range of values and variables to determine when it is maximally functional. When the variables and values are identified, they can be compared to the variables noted by the respondents to determine how well they match.

Other procedures for establishing competency norms have been offered (Kazdin, 1977c; Van Houten, 1979). It is recognized, however, that the process is a long and perhaps arduous one seldom accomplished by a single experimenter or in a short period. Rather, it requires a long-term commitment with a variety of investigators participating in accumulation of information on variables involved in many behaviors until eventually standards of competency are derived to which treatment efforts can be directed.

The other method for measuring social importance is subjective evaluation. In principle, it involves using expert judges to rate the behavior of subjects before and after treatment (Kazdin, 1977c). It is possible to use community members as in the Jones and Azrin (1969) study, clients themselves as in the Braukmann et al. (1976) study, or a panel of expert judges for the rating. Sometimes ratings are made of the behavior alone, but often this entails a more global judgment of the subjects' behavioral repertoire in an environmental setting.

Many of the criteria discussed thus far for evaluating treatment effectiveness pertain to graphic analysis or visual inspection of data. However, statistical analysis of data is gaining in popularity and presents other criteria. The next section is devoted to a brief overview for use of statistical criteria.

STATISTICAL CRITERIA FOR EVALUATING TREATMENT EFFECTIVENESS

Behavior analysts have employed clinical and experimental criteria to assess treatment effectiveness (Kazdin, 1977c). Clinical criterion, the less objective of the two, developed from the belief that applied research should be restricted to topics that are of clinical or social importance (Baer, Wolf, and Risley, 1968). In applying this philosophy, applied researchers have pursued large, clinically significant changes in behavior and small, less obvious treatment effects have been viewed as less important. Emphasis on clinical criterion is also reflected in attempts to obtain social validation of experimental findings. The second criterion employed by applied researchers, experimental criterion, refers to the treatment, no-treatment comparison which is inherent in both within-subject and group study paradigms. The primary experimental criteria in within-subject research has been visual analysis of data, whereas inferential statistics have served as the predominant means of evaluating group study data. Increasingly, however, the reliability of visual analysis procedures is being questioned and inferential statistics are being proposed as alternative or supplementary criteria for assessing within-subject findings (DeProspero and Cohen, 1979; Jones et al., 1978; Wampold and Furlong, 1981). In particular, tests of significance have been proposed as a means of establishing the reliability (believability) of within-subject findings when visual analysis is inconclusive (Browning, 1967; Edgington, 1967; Gentile et al., 1972; Jones et al., 1977; Revusky, 1967). Visual analysis procedures may prove inconclusive when treatment effects are small or intrasubject variability is large. Similarly, complex changes in the slope and/or level of data may also preclude unambiguous visual interpretation. Yet, despite the limitations of visual analysis, actual use of inferential statistics in the within-subject literature has been limited (Kratochwill and Brody, 1978).

The purpose of this section is to discuss the rationale for continued use of visual analysis as the primary experimental criterion for within-subject studies and to highlight the controversy surrounding the use of statistics in applied research. Applied investigators have disavowed inferential statistics because their use is not consistent with several basic tenets of the behavorial analytic philosophy and because proposed statistics do not easily accommodate the unique problems associated with time-series data. Each of these factors is considered in the following discussion.

Failure to Meet Statistical Assumptions

From a technical standpoint, few inferential statistical methods are well suited to within-subject studies because important statistical assumptions about characteristics of data are seldom met in time-series research. Moreover, serious violations of the assumptions that underly tests of significance invalidate or considerably limit inferences that can be drawn from a statistical analysis. Foremost among the assumptions that must be met for proper application of statistics is the independence assumption, which states that extraneous influences on a variable must be both random and independent. Whereas independence of error factors may be assumed in many group studies for which inferential statistics were originally intended, this assumption is rarely met in within-subject studies. Applied behavorial data are collected frequently over time and from the same subject. As a result, scores tend to be "serially dependent" rather than independent (Revusky, 1967; Johnston and Pennypacker, 1980; Jones et al., 1977). That is, contrary to the independence assumption, within-subject scores are influenced by, and to a certain extent, predictive of one another. Given this, variations of traditional statistics, such as Gentile, Roden, and Klein's (1972) analysis of variance procedure, are not appropriate for use in within-subject research (Hartmann, 1974; Jones et al., 1977). Other methods that have been suggested to avoid the problems posed by serial dependence involve the random assignment of experimental phases before statistical evaluation of treatment effectiveness (Edgington, 1967; Revusky, 1967). Although these procedures do, in fact, satisfy the assumption of statistical independence, practical shortcomings of randomization methods may delimit their use (Kazdin, 1976). In addition, the practice of designing experiments primarily on the basis of statistical considerations is objectionable because this approach removes flexibility and, to a certain extent, ingenuity from the investigative process.

To date, only one statistical method adequately circumvents the problem of serial dependence in applied behavorial research. Labeled *interrupted time series analysis* (ITSA), this approach determines the degree of serial dependence between scores obtained over time, transforms scores to a serially independent state, and then statistically compares between phase differences in level, trend, and change in data trends (Jones et al., 1977). This unique analysis procedure has been proposed as a powerful supplement to visual analysis when treatment effects are difficult to discern visually. For example, Jones et al. (1977) demonstrated that time-series analysis is applicable to basic within-subject designs and may provide information over and above that obtained through visual analysis alone. It is important to note, however, that visual analysis and interrupted time-series analysis may not lead to the same inferences, particularly when data are highly serially dependent (Jones et al., 1978) and such discrepancies may be difficult to reconcile. One might be tempted to rely on results obtained through the time series analysis because of the presumed objectivity of statistical procedures. Bakan (1966) reminds us, however, that statistics ''...can serve to obscure as well as reveal'' (p. 436). It would not be prudent to dismiss conclusions based on visual analysis simply because they are discrepant with inferences reached through time series or any other statistical procedure. Unlike visual analysis, time series analysis has seldom been used in behavior analytic research and the limitations of this approach are relatively unknown. Hartmann et al. (1980) indicate that time series analysis may prove to be more reliable than visual analysis of serially dependent data, particularly when visual effects of treatment are not obvious. They also note however, that ''...with time series that include few observations, particularly those in which visual analysis indicate a treatment effect which is not supported by the results of ITSA, greater credence may be given to the results of the visual analysis'' (p. 555). From a practical standpoint it is noteworthy that time series analysis is technically complex and, in fact, a computer is needed to complete the analysis. Consequently, the benefits of time series analysis may not be available to the majority of clinical researchers who are not likely to have access to the technical assistance or hardware necessary to conduct the analysis.

Over and above their failure to meet important assumptions, statistical data have also been criticized because they have frequently been misused and misinterpreted (Bakan, 1966; Carver, 1978). Abuse and practical limitations aside, however, appropriate statistical procedures are available for within-subject research (Jones et al., 1977; Kazdin, 1976) and these problems have not been the primary deterrent to adoption of statistical criteria. More salient arguments against the use of statistics have arisen from applied researchers who believe that statistical criteria are not consistent with the philosophy and aims of applied behavioral research (Baer et al., 1968; Michael, 1974b; Baer, 1977b). As Kazdin (1976) notes, ''whether statistical analysis *should* be used to evaluate change in intra-subject replication designs has been a major point of contention'' (p. 265). Philosophical objections to the use of statistics as experimental criteria for within-subject research is considered in the following section.

Behavior-Analytic Objections to Inferential Statistics

One reason that statistics has been viewed as inapplicable to applied research is that the logic of inferential statistics accepts inter- or intrasubject variability as inevitable and places chance in a nearly sacrosanct position. When tests of significance are employed, a null hypothesis is stated which assumes that intergroup or intrasubject differences are due to random variability or sampling error. That is, it is hypothesized that there is no 'true' difference between treatment and no-treatment conditions. Tests of significance let us calculate the probability of getting obtained results if they were due to chance variability. If the calculated probability (P level) is small, usually below 5 %, then the null hypothesis of no difference is rejected because the obtained results would rarely be expected on the basis of chance alone. Statistical procedures are also used to "control" known variables that might affect research findings. A major criticism of this general approach is that it de-emphasizes the need experimentally to control unwanted variability. As Sidman (1960) states,

> To some experimenters, chance is simply a name for the combined effects of uncontrolled variables. If such variables are, in fact, controllable, then chance in this sense is simply an excuse for sloppy experimentation, and no further comment is required. If the uncontrolled variables are actually unknown, then chance is . . . a synonym for ignorance. Science is presumably dedicated to stamping out ignorance, but statistical evaluation of data against a baseline whose characteristics are determined by unknown variables constitutes a passive acceptance of ignorance. This is a curious negation of the professed aims of science. More consistent with those aims is the evaluation of data by means of experimental control . . . (p. 45)

As this quote emphasizes, Sidman (1960) proposes that applied researchers discover and control sources of variability rather than assume that variability is intrinsic to their subjects. Intense within-subject designs permit an evaluation of functional relationships between behavior and environmental conditions that may contribute to variability. If excessive intrasubject variability is evident, then investigators should search for the source and bring it under control. Tests of significance do not remove or 'control' unwanted variability. They simply let us infer whether uncontrolled variables contributed to an experimental outcome.

A second major objection to statistics relates to our previous discussion of clinical and experimental criteria. As we noted earlier, statistical procedures have been advocated for use in within-subject research when treatment effects are equivocal through visual analysis. When visual analysis is inconclusive, statistics can be used to tease out subtle treatment effects. The question arises, however, whether subtle effects are worth discovering. Recall that many applied researchers are only concerned with large, clinically significant changes and smaller changes revealed through statistical analysis may be viewed as unimportant. The discovery of powerful variables that effect large changes in behavior is consistent with both the subject matter and basic philosophy of applied behavior analysis. Applied researchers are likely to be involved in attempting to solve an immediate clinical problem that requires marked changes in behavior and the discovery of factors that have little influence on behavior is often uninteresting. Take, for example, the case of a severe stutterer who suffers considerable embarrassment or social and professional restrictions because of his communicative handicap. Discovery of a treatment that provides a minor reduction in disfluency rate may be of academic interest. However, the ultimate goal of an applied study of this individual's communication problem would probably be to increase his fluency to a near normal rate. Consequently, the results of a within-subject study would be considered clinically significant if the change in fluency rate was marked and visually obvious. Alternately, an improvement that was small and had to be teased out statistically might be considered a mere curiosity. Baer (1977b) distinguished between the types of results discovered through statistics and those revealed through visual analysis as follows. He stated, statistics "...will uncover a host of weak, occasional, or otherwise highly specialized variables" (p. 170); whereas visual analysis reveals variables that "...are typically more powerful, general, dependable, and—very important—sometimes actionable" (p. 171).

Time spent on statistical analysis will, no doubt, reveal numerous subtle variables that could be further researched for their therapeutic potential. It is, however, the discovery of large treatment effects that have an immediate impact on a client's communicative disorder that is most consistent with the goals of applied behavioral research. In addition, the discovery of powerful and immediately useful variables will lead to a more rapidly developing science of human behavior (Johnston and Pennypacker, 1980). Despite common assumptions, statistically significant results are not necessarily important or replicable (Bakan, 1966; Carver, 1978). For a given study, inferences based on statistical analysis are only reliable in a probabalistic sense. Failure to obtain replication of statistically significant findings may occur under the most ideal conditions because relatively small differences may be "significant." Unfortunately, publication of results that are statistically significant may actually inhibit replication attempts and discourage investigators from submitting studies that do not reach an arbitrary level of significance (Bakan, 1966; Rosenthal, 1979). The lack of direct or systematic replications in the communicative disorders literature, a literature that has adhered to the group study, inferential statistics paradigms, appears to support this contention, and the seriousness of this problem cannot be overlooked. As Smith (1970) noted "...if the goal of scientific research is to render established truths, then the neglect of replication must be viewed as scientific irresponsibility" (p. 971).

Unlike statistical criteria, the use of visual analysis and search for large treatment effects encourages replication attempts. Within-subject research designs actually incorporate replication into their procedures by repeatedly applying and removing an independent variable within a given subject over time. In addition, replication of within-subject findings across subjects has become standard practice and a basic requirement for publication of single-case experimental studies. Because some variability in responding can be expected within and across subjects, "replication is the essence of believability" (Baer et al., 1968, p. 95). As in group study research, reliance on statistics may give behavior analysts a false sense of security about their data and this, in turn, could have the adverse effect of discouraging replication attempts. At the present time, visual analysis encourages the search for treatment variables that are sufficiently large and unequivocal. Moreover, because visually obvious effects result from powerful variables, attempted replications are likely to be successful. Thus, maintaining traditional visual rather than statistical analysis may foster the technical advancement of clinical sciences, such as in the field of communicative disorders.

One final reason why applied behavioral researchers have shunned statistics is worthy of brief consideration. Michael (1974b) reminds us that both visual and statistical analysis procedures are "judgment aids" designed to facilitate data interpretation. He points out, however, that statistical procedures result in abbreviations of raw data that reduce the amount of information available for analysis. Statistics may, in fact, simplify the interpretation by dichotomizing the effects of treatment as significant or nonsignificant. The desirability of the simplification process is, however, open to question. Within-subject research is a deliberate departure from the group study, statistical analysis paradigm. The fine-grain analysis characteristic of this approach requires detailed and ongoing analysis, and a return to a statistical model will, no doubt, diminish the intensity of the inferential process. Even if graphic and statistical analyses were presented together (Jones et al., 1977; Hartmann et al., 1980), there would be an ever-present danger of "accepting" or emphasizing statistically significant results when visual analysis proved inconclusive. For example, manuscripts that emphasized statistical results might have a better chance of being published in journals that use statistics as a criteria for publication and thus, in turn, would reinforce the use of and reliance on statistics. In any event, as Michael (1974b) notes, "...whether by necessity, scientific cunning, or prejudice, operant researchers, basic and applied, have made little use of statistical inference and do not seem to have suffered as a result. Increasingly sophisticated methods of experimental control have developed within the area of basic research, and applied researchers have generally been able to make use of the same technology, or develop methods of experimental control appropriate to their own problems" (pp. 650–651).

SUMMARY

Data directly related to the behavior studied forms the core data base from which treatment results are evaluated. Criteria for evaluating relevance of the data to the problem at hand include both within- and across-phase factors. In general, visual inspection seeks to determine if the trend, slope, and level of data points within and across phases provide clear evidence of changes as conditions alternate during the experiment.

Criteria for evaluating treatment effectiveness are not confined to within experimental data. Indeed, evidence of generality must be offered before a treatment is considered successful. Generality is established through replications. Direct replications establish generality of the treatment to other individuals similar to the subjects involved in the studies. Systematic replications confirm generality of the treatment to other subjects, in other situations, and in the presence of more than one experimenter administering the treatment. Clinical replication examines the effectiveness of a treatment package composed of elements that have been identified in previous studies. After a series of single-subject designs in which single independent variables have been evaluated and their generality confirmed in direct and systematic replications, the variables may be compiled into a treatment program to be administered to groups of clients. Study of individual components is called technique building and testing entire treatment packages is technique testing. The latter falls into the category of clinical replication. The final step in evaluating effectiveness of treatment is determining if the behavior changes are socially valid. Several procedures are used to determine whether the changes are appropriate enough to satisfy not only the client but other individuals who come in daily contact with the subject. Thus, if social importance of the behavioral change can be established, the final criterion for treatment effectiveness is attained.

Statistical criteria for evaluating treatment effectiveness are gaining wider use among within-subject researchers. Possibly, single-subject statistics will become common in experimental analysis research. Nevertheless, use of inferential statistics presents problems regarding sampling and generality. Recognizing the shortcomings of inferential statistics, most behavior analysts choose to depend on replications for evidence of generality.

Reliability and Observational Codes

5

It should be apparent from the information in the preceding chapter that evaluation of therapeutic effectiveness in within-subject research is a complex and challenging process. In addition to considering previously discussed criteria for evaluating behavior change, the investigator must also be aware of confounding elements that might affect the data. For example, applied behavioral research frequently depends on human observers to record subject behavior; yet perceptual judgments are subject to error and variability, and factors such as idiosyncratic scoring and examiner bias affect recording of observational data. Investigators cannot, therefore, assume that observer recordings are accurate. Thus reliability, the primary means of evaluating accuracy and objectivity of observer-recorded data, is also an important criterion for evaluating believability of single-subject research data.

The term *reliability* generally refers to consistency and reproducibility of observation and measurement (Thorndike and Hagen, 1977). Although there are numerous approaches to measuring reliability, this discussion is restricted to the interjudge agreement method, the most prevalent found in single-subject intervention literature (Kelly, 1977).

To determine interjudge reliability, two or more independent and unbiased judges simultaneously record target responses according to predetermined operational definitions and a scoring code. After a period of observation, the observer recordings are compared and a percentage agreement score is calculated. High levels of interjudge agreement (reliability) are taken as an indication that the observer accurately recorded the behavior of interest. That is, independent confirmation is provided indicating that the data reflect a true change in subject behavior rather than variability in observer recording. As Hawkins and Farby (1979) note, we are likely to inquire ''Is that what I would have seen had I been there?'' when we are evaluating data. High levels of interobserver reliability allow us to conclude with greater confidence that our observations would have been consistent with these reported.

Failure to obtain consistent and reproducible levels of interjudge agreement leaves an investigator in the position of being unable to interpret the data. Take for example the situation in which low levels of agreement are reached between two observers of the same behavior, and one observer records a significant improvement in the subject's performance during an intervention phase but a second does not. When this occurs, the only conclusion that can be reached is that one or both of the observers incorrectly tallied the target behavior.

As we have seen, very high or very low levels of reliability are not problematic. Interpretive difficulty arises, however, when reliability coefficients lie between these extreme levels. A relevant consideration, therefore, is what constitutes an "acceptable" level of interobserver agreement. Although percentages of 80% to 100% may be considered satisfactory for some observational data, it is difficult to establish specific guidelines for minimally acceptable levels of agreement (Kazdin, 1977a, b). For example, factors such as complexity of the behavioral coding system, number of reliability checks conducted, influence of artifacts and bias, and the method used to calculate the reliability coefficient must be considered in assessing reliability and these cannot be standardized.

Although specific criteria cannot be established for "acceptable" reliability, this does not diminish its prominent role in applied research. It seems difficult, in fact, to overestimate the importance of reliable measurement in human experimentation. As Neale and Liebert (1973) note, "...the first and most important aspect of collecting useful information is reliable measurement" (p. 87). Ironically, evidence in the applied behavioral literature indicates that researchers may have underestimated the complexity of reliability measurement and calculation. Interobserver agreement may not provide a sensitive index of the objectivity of behavioral recordings. Observers may, for example, agree that a subject responded at a given level when, in fact, he did not, or, conversely, an experimenter may accurately record behavior but not achieve a high level of agreement with an independent observer (Bijou, Peterson and Ault, 1968; Hawkins and Dotson, 1975). The remainder of this chapter considers factors that may have an important effect on measurement, calculation, or interpretation of interjudge reliability data. In addition, special consideration will be given to factors particularly relevant to single-subject intervention research in communicative disorders.

PRE-EXPERIMENTAL CONSIDERATIONS

Prior to initiation of an intervention study an investigator makes several decisions that may have a significant effect on the reliability of the data. The investigator must, for example, operationally define the behaviors of interest, develop a corresponding scoring code, and select an appropriate method for data collection. These preexperimental decisions are, of course, based on individual considerations of the type, frequency, and complexity of the behavior under examination; quantitative guidelines cannot be established to assist investigators in making these important decisions. Nonetheless, several related considerations reviewed in this section may prove beneficial to the investigator who is planning the reliability phase of a study.

Operational Definitions

One of the most important aspects of the proposal phase of an investigation is operationally defining the behaviors of interest. Inadequate response definitions may result in unacceptable levels of interobserver agreement and thereby invalidate experimental results. As Bijou et al. (1968) note, "Observer reliability is directly related to the comprehensiveness and specificity of definitions in the observational code" (p. 183).

In order to be considered operational, response definitions should be comprehensive, specific, and mutually exclusive. That is, each behavior should be defined in such a way that it clearly specifies which events will be included in a response category and which will not. In addition, there should be no overlap between response categories. Definitions that are overly inclusive do not delineate important from unimportant behaviors, and make it difficult to evaluate or replicate experimental findings. In addition, observer disagreements may result from an inadequately specified behavioral code. Therefore, when low levels of reliability are obtained, the investigator should closely examine response definitions to determine their contribution to lack of observer agreement.

The following example from the communicative disorders literature demonstrates the level of specificity required for an operational response definition. Reid and Hurlbut (1977) reported a multiple-baseline study examining the effects of a training program on use of a communication board by physically handicapped retarded adults. Four subjects were individually trained to point to word-picture combinations on the board in response to verbal descriptions provided by the examiners. Three of the subjects used head pointers to respond, and the fourth pointed with his hand. Because the number of correct selections on the communication board was the dependent variable in this study, it was necessary to define carefully which pointing responses would be considered correct and which would not. Therefore, the following response definition was provided by Reid and Hurlbut (1977): "A correct point was defined as the end of the head pointer (or the most protruding portion of the hand . . .) stopping within the border lines of the block on the communication board designed by the trainer. The pointer, or hand, had to touch the board without movement within the block for a minimum of 1 second and had to occur within 10 seconds of the trainer's request" (p. 593).

Although relatively specific, it should be noted that this definition by itself would not have been operational. It would not, for example, indicate how a self correction would have been scored, or which response would have been tallied if multiple responses were produced. Thus, the authors also specified their definition of an error response as follows: "1) the end of pointer (or hand...) stopping on any part of the board for a minimum of 1 second except the trainer's designated block or 2) end of the pointer (or hand) not stopping on any part of the board for a minimum of 1 second within 10 seconds of a trainer's request. If the subject pointed to two or more blocks for a minimum of 1 second each within 10 seconds of a trainer's request, the first block pointed to determined whether the response was correct or incorrect." (p. 593).

The definition of an incorrect pointing response helped to clarify any ambiguity that might have occurred had the authors relied exclusively on the definition of a correct pointing response. Thus, when combined, the correct and incorrect definitions appear to provide an operational definition for the pointing responses in this study. Moreover, this conclusion is supported by the levels of interobserver agreement reported for the identification training phase of this study (93% to 100%). It should be cautioned, however, that although interobserver reliability provides an index of the acceptability of operational definitions, high levels of observer agreement alone do not ensure that response definitions are sufficiently specific or complete (Hawkins and Dotson, 1975).

One final comment on the response definitions in this example appears relevant. Recall that Reid and Hurlbut (1977) specified the location and duration of an acceptable pointing response and the time frame within which the response would be considered correct, and identified which response would be scored when multiple responses were produced. It should be noted that deletion of any of these components might have affected the obtained levels of interobserver agreement. For example, disagreements could have resulted between the experimenter and an observer if one had scored only first responses and the second scored only the last. Similarly, exclusion of any components of the definition of a pointing response could have resulted in interpretive difficulties, despite high levels of interobserver agreement. For example, even though the experimenter and an independent observer agreed that a subject's pointing response was correct on a given trial, we could not be certain that they had scored the same response if the authors had not indicated that only the first of multiple responses would be scored. Thus, it is imperative that all relevant dimensions of a response be clearly specified if acceptable levels of interobserver agreement are to be reached, and meaningful interpretation of reliability calculations is to be possible.

Direct Measurement Techniques

Before proceeding with our discussion of observational codes and interobserver agreement, it may be beneficial to reconsider briefly earlier comments about the type of data generally obtained in within-subject investigations. It will be recalled that a basic requirement of applied behavioral research is that target behaviors should be directly observable. That is, indirect measurements interpreted as being representative of underlying thoughts, states, or feelings are eschewed for carefully defined, directly observable responses. For example, indirect measures of anxiety or personality characteristics of dysfluent subjects would be seen as tangential to the problem of modifying stuttering. In contrast, following the direct measurement approach, target behaviors (e.g., phoneme repetitions) would be carefully defined, recorded, and subsequently targeted for treatment. As Hersen and Barlow (1976) note, "Under the system of direct measurement rates of specified behaviors within designated time periods may be used as dependent measures during pre-treatment assessment (and) actual treatment..." (p. 117). They further note that measurements such as having subjects monitor and report their own behavior are subject to willful distortion and bias and may be of limited use as dependent variables in treatment research.

A review of observational data collection and reliability procedures in the *Journal of Applied Behavior Analysis* by Kelly (1977) reveals that 76% of the 293 studies reported from 1968 through 1975 presented direct observational data, 16% reported only mechanically recorded data, and the remaining 8% of the studies reported only permanent product data (e.g., written responses). It is apparent from the results that the human observer remains the primary measurement instrument in applied behavior analytic research. However, in the following section we review each of the common types of observational codes or data collection procedures used in single-subject research because the method of data collection may have a considerable effect on the reliability of data collected.

OBSERVATIONAL CODES

An observational code refers to the method of scoring and recording behaviors the investigator has operationally defined and plans to investigate. A code may range from a simple check mark on a piece of paper when the behavior is observed to an elaborate symbol system that identifies a variety of possible responses produced by a given subject. As noted above, electromechanical, observational, and permanent product data collection procedures may be used to code and/or record behavioral data.

Electromechanical Recording

Although less frequently used than observer coding procedures (Kelly, 1977), instrumental recording of human behavior has several advantages over other methods of data collection. For example, error and bias, which may occur when humans record data, are greatly diminished when automated procedures are employed. In addition, electromechanical data recording has the potential to record accurately temporal aspects of subject behavior, to automatically monitor a large number of responses, and may require less of an investigator's time than other procedures (Bijou et al., 1968). Despite these advantages, however, it is not surprising that a relatively small proportion of applied studies rely exclusively on instrumental data collection. Instrumental recording is more expensive and less flexible than use of human observers. In addition, the high frequency of studies in naturalistic settings and the diversity of behaviors observed often preclude use of electromechanical data collection.

Automated Quantitative Recording Procedures

Hersen and Barlow (1976) have dichotomized instrumental recording of behavior into "automated quantitative" and "non-automated quantitative" methods. Automated quantitative procedures are those in which "apparatus consisting of electronic circuitry is connected to cumulative recorders" (p. 120), and the behavior of interest is automatically tallied as soon as it occurs. Although use of completely automated recording procedures is infrequent in studies of communicative disorders, examples of this approach can be found in the literature. A previously discussed study by Roll (1973), for example, employed an automated quantitative data recording system. The purpose was to investigate the effects of differential visual feedback on the amount of hypernasality produced by cleft palate children. The apparatus used to record instances of hypernasality consisted of an electromechanical transducer, a voice-operated relay system, and an electronically operated digital counter. Each time a subject produced a response, the transducer recorded the amount of vibration in his nasal cavity (hypernasality). Responses that vibrated the nasal cavity above a predetermined level (i.e., those that were hypernasal) were transduced into electrical energy and activated the voice-operated relay system. In turn, the relay system triggered the digital recorder, which automatically recorded the response. Thus, each response was immediately and automatically coded as hypernasal or non-nasal and counted. That is, the experimenter was not directly involved in the data collection process.

Several interesting aspects of this study deserve further mention. First, interobserver reliability was not reported in this study because each response was automatically recorded. That is, the author assumed that the equipment reliably recorded each response as either nasalized or non-nasalized. The author was, however, cognizant of the need to ensure that the data accurately reflected change in the subject's behavior. For example, the amount of nasality recorded might reflect alternate sites of placement of the transducer rather than a real change in the subject's speech. Care was taken, therefore, to use the same procedure for transducer placement before each session, and to recalibrate sensitivity of the relay system.

As the above precautions indicate, use of automated quantitative measurement procedures does not relieve the investigator of the responsibility to ensure that the data are reliable. Frequent calibration of the apparatus and recording procedures should be an integral component of such studies. Moreover, as we shall see in our discussion of nonautomated quantitive procedures, use of instrumentation does not necessarily eliminate need for interobserver reliability measurements.

Nonautomated Quantitative Recording

There are several advantages and disadvantages in observational and instrumental recording of data in applied research. As already noted, although human observers may be less expensive and more flexible than instrumental measurement procedures, they are also more prone to scoring variability and bias than their electromechanical counterparts. Alternately, although automated quantitative measurement procedures are likely to be more reliable than human observers, they may have limited application in naturalistic settings or when diverse behaviors are being coded. They require programming or electronic knowledge to operate and are more expensive than human observer-recorders. An investigator is not, however, restricted to these choices when deciding upon an appropriate measurement tool for a given study. Occasionally, the limitations of automated quantitative and observer recording procedures can be overcome by measuring the rate or level of behavior on a standard scale or instrument, and then relying on humans to read and record the obtained data. Labeled a *nonautomated quantitative* approach, this method is relatively free from human error or bias because human participation is restricted to recording aspects of data collection, and perceptual judgments are minimized (Hersen and Barlow, 1976). Several instruments are available for clinical research in communicative disorders which may be considered nonautomated, quantitative methods of data collection. For example, a commercially available instrument that provides a continuous digital readout of fundamental frequency (Fletcher, 1972) is nonautomated and quantitative in nature because an experimenter using it must read the frequency level displayed and then record it on appropriate data sheets. A second example from the communicative disorders literature is briefly described in the following section.

Jackson and Wallace (1974) examined the effects of a token-based treatment program on the vocal intensity of a young subject with a habitually low loudness level. Details of this study have been previously presented in Chapter 2 and the present discussion is restricted to the method of data collection and reliability procedures employed. It will be recalled that tokens were automatically delivered contingent upon production of target words at a specified loudness level during the treatment phases of this investigation. Measurement and recording of the dependent variable, vocal intensity, was not, however, totally automated. Rather, a ''decibel meter'' was used to monitor the subject's intensity level and the ''experimenter recorded the intensity of each response, measured as the extent of the needle deflection on the decibel meter'' (p. 463). The data were reported as the average loudness levels obtained during shaping and generalization sessions. Thus, the experimenter's role in the data collection procedures involved reading and recording intensity levels measured on the sound level meter, and subsequently averaging these measurements. Therefore, a nonautomated, quantitative data collection procedure was utilized.

It should be noted that although use of standard measuring instruments, such as a sound level meter, may reduce the opportunity for human error in nonautomated, quantitative data collection procedures, this opportunity is not eliminated. Whenever possible, the investigator should report interobserver reliability for those aspects of the measurement procedure that involved human participation. In the Jackson and Wallace (1974) study, for example, one would expect some variability in reading points of maximal needle deflection on the sound level meter. Recognizing this, the authors had an independent observer measure the loudness of selected speech samples with the decibel meter so that these measurements could be compared with the experimenter's and a level of interobserver agreement computed. Further confidence could, therefore, be placed in the findings of this study because evidence was provided indicating the data were reliable.

Several additional aspects of the data collection and reliability procedures utilized in this investigation are of interest. For instance, although interobserver agreement data were presented, closer examination reveals that reported agreement was for ''lab generalization'' sessions, not for the ''shaping,'' or treatment, phase of the study. Given that different reading tasks were presented in each of these experimental conditions, it might have been beneficial if interobserver agreement had also been reported for the treatment portion of the investigation so that the contribution of scoring variability could be evaluated. This would seem particularly crucial in studies such as this one, in which relatively small changes in the dependent variable are reported (see Figure 6).

Finally, examination of the reliability data in this study reveals that interobserver agreement calculations were based on average readings of the decibel meter. That is, an average loudness level per word was computed from 50 word-reading samples, the mean loudness level per word obtained by the experimenter and reliability judge was compared, and percentage agreement scores obtained. The pitfalls of mean data have been previously discussed, and there is no need to elaborate here. Given the relatively small increase in loudness level needed for the subject to match performance of her normal peers, however, mean data should have been avoided so that the absolute difference and amount of variability present in the recordings could have been evaluated for each session for which reliability was obtained. Average data disguises variability that may be present and does not permit an unequivocal evaluation of reported results.

It should be apparent from the above discussion that a careful consideration of the relationship between the data collection procedure and reliability of the data is a necessary component of applied research even when nonautomated quantitative measurement techniques are employed. In the following review of data collection procedures that rely on human observers as the primary measurement instrument, we explore the relationship between methods of observation, observational codes, and interobserver reliability.

OBSERVATIONAL MEASUREMENT

The rapid development of microcircuitry may be expected to increase significantly the use of instrumentation in the rehabilitative field (Holbrook, 1980). In communicative disorders various forms of physiologically based instrumentally recorded feedback have, for example, been employed in attempts to modify the behavior of subjects with dysarthria and voice and fluency disorders (Netsell and Cleeland, 1973; Holbrook, 1980; Hanna, Wilfing, and McNeill, 1975) and this trend toward increasing use of instrumentation in clinical research may be expected to continue. Human observers are presently the primary measurement instrument in applied behavioral research (Kelly, 1977), however, and it is unlikely that they will be replaced by electromechanical recording devices in the near future. Ironically, selection of an observational code is currently a highly individualized and somewhat arbitrary process (Kent and Foster, 1977). Furthermore, the choice is a complicated one based on a number of considerations that do not permit the establishment of specific criteria. As Kazdin (1977a, b) points out, "the method of assessment employed is dictated by such factors as the goals of investigation, the specific response observed, the rate of responding, the ease with which responses can be detected, and a variety of practical ex- igencies. While some responses appear to be more readily assessed by a par- ticular method, alternate methods are usually available" (p. 67).

Despite the myriad of factors that must be considered, selection of an appropriate observational code is prerequisite to reliable data collection and investigators must be familiar with available data-collection techniques. Therefore, frequently employed observational codes will be reviewed and related to communicative disorders literature in the discussion that follows. Specifically, the following categories of codes reviewed by Kelly (1977) in his survey of the data collection procedures in the *Journal of Applied Behavior Analysis* will be considered:

1. Trial scoring (used in 35% of the studies surveyed)
2. Event recording (29%)
3. Time sampling (21%)
4. Interval recording (20%), and
5. Response duration (9%)

Trial Scoring

Trial scoring or the recording of a response as correct or incorrect following a specific stimulus or experimenal trial, accounts for a large number of applied studies in communicative disorders. (Bennett, 1974; Clark and Sherman, 1975; Garcia, 1974; Hegde, Noll, and Pecora, 1979; Reid and Hurlbut, 1977). Frisch and Schumaker (1974) employed trial-by-trial scoring in their procedure for training receptive language skills in retarded children. A multiple-baseline design across behaviors was used to train three categories of prepositional requests (put "x" next to /under/ on top of "y"). During the baseline phase the experimenter placed an object of the preposition (e.g., a bucket) directly in front of a subject, handed him a direct object (e.g., a shovel), and then stated a prepositional request (e.g., "Put the shovel next to the bucket"). No feedback or consequation was provided during this phase. During the training phase of the study, commands for the target prepositions were presented and verbal feedback, tangible rewards, and prompts were used to shape appropriate responding. After successfully training the first prepositonal category, the remaining categories were sequentially trained.

Throughout each phase of this study, each response was scored as correct or incorrect according to predetermined operational definitions. Thus, Frisch and Schumaker (1974) state that "a correct response to a 'next to' request was recorded when the subject placed the direct object (the item handed him by the experimenter) on the table within 1 inch (2.5 cm) of the object of the preposition "the item on the table" (p. 614). All other "next to" responses and any absence of response within 10 seconds of the stimulus presentation were scored incorrect. Interobserver reliability was evaluated by having an observer in the room during selected training and probe sessions from each phase of the study. Interobserver agreement was calculated by comparing the observer's and the experimenter's scoring on a trial-by-trial basis.

In addition to trial-by-trial recording of the accuracy of responding, numerous other forms of discrete trial scoring have been reported in the literature. These include phonetic or word-for-word transcription, the use of symbols or codes to represent categories of responses, and numerical codes (Bennett, 1974; Clark and Sherman, 1975; Garcia, 1974; Mann and Baer, 1971; Schreibman and Carr, 1978). Combinations of these observational codes, and correct/incorrect scoring of multiple behaviors after a single experimental trial, have also been reported.

Perhaps the greatest advantage of trial-by-trial scoring is its relative simplicity because higher levels of interobserver agreement can be expected for less complex observational codes (Mash and McElwee, 1974; Kent and Foster, 1977). Thus, one might expect higher levels of reliability for studies using a correct/incorrect scoring code for a single behavior as opposed to those employing trial-by-trial scoring of multiple behaviors. As we shall see in our discussion of the influence of chance agreement on reliability calculation, however, higher coefficients of agreement that result from use of simpler observation codes do not guarantee that observer recordings are accurate. Moreover, the simplicity of trial-by-trial recording may be deceiving, particularly when scoring procedures are employed that indirectly represent the behaviors under investigation. An example of such a code is presented in the following discussion.

Numerical Coding Procedures

Numerical coding procedures provide a potentially efficient means of recording a subject's behaviors. An investigator can, for example, develop a numerical code in which a single number represents several dimensions of responding. As Porch (1971) notes, plus-minus scoring captures the accuracy of responding, but other valuable information may be omitted. Although an experimenter could supplement plus-minus scoring systems with written notes on a subject's behavior, this procedure is cumbersome and unsystematic and does not, therefore, offer a useful alternative. Multidimensional scoring codes, however, provide reasonable alternatives to correct/incorrect scoring.

The use of a multidimensional scoring code involves representing several basic dimensions of responding with a single number. Porch (1971), for example, developed a sixteen-point scoring scale for recording the responses of aphasic clients. Each number in the scale represents combinations of five dimensions (accuracy, responsiveness, completeness, promptness, and efficiency) he felt were necessary for adequately describing aphasic patient's attempts to communicate. Higher numbers in the system are used to describe responses that include increasingly more of these characteristics, and subtle distinctions in responding can be represented using this numerical code. Thus, a score of "15" represents a response that is "complete" according to the given dimensional system and a score of "13" is assigned to responses that are complete following a delay.

Although multidimensional scoring procedures provide a potentially efficient and comprehensive manner of recording communicative behaviors, their use has been primarily restricted to diagnostic testing (Porch, 1971; McNeil and Prescott, 1978). The complexity of these scoring systems have limited their availability to individuals who have received extensive training and practice with the codes. Thus, as in the case with other complex observational codes, the potential benefits they offer an investigator must be weighed against the practical necessity for reliability training. In addition, although comprehensive numerical codes have potential for efficiently communicating experimental findings to individuals familiar with the scoring procedure, research consumers not familiar with the code may be limited by their inability to interpret results of studies that use them.

In addition to multidimensional scoring, other types of numerical coding procedures have been reported in the communicative disorders literature. For example, codes have been reported in which each number in the system represents a particular response type. Rosenbaum and Breiling (1976) employed a five-point rating scale in their investigation of a remedial procedure for training reading comprehension skills. The subject of this study, an autistic child, was asked to read and follow simple motor commands (e.g., "stand up"; "point to the ball") printed on cue cards. During the treatment phase, edibles, verbal praise, and prompts, modeling, and physical guidance were used to train the subject to follow the printed commands. Of primary interest to this discussion was the scoring code. A score of 5 was recorded if the subject performed the printed instructions within 10 seconds of stimulus presentation. Scores of 4, 3, or 2, respectively, were assigned to responses that were correct after a verbal prompt, a model of the response, or physical guidance. A score of 1 was recorded for responses that were incorrect despite the above attempts to prompt the subject. Thus, unlike multidimensional scoring codes in which a single number indicates that a behavior consisted of several predetermined response dimensions, the code employed in this study represented the type of experimenter cue that preceded each response. A single score was indicative of each response type.

As previously noted, an important consideration in evaluating data represented by a numerical code is whether numbers within the scoring system directly represent the behavior of interest. The interpretive difficulties that can arise when numerical codes are employed are demonstrated in the following example.

Garcia (1974) used a composite numerical code while examining effects of differential consequation and imitation on the verbal production of target sentences by two nonverbal, retarded children. The subjects were trained to produce target sentences in response to pictorial and verbal stimuli. After reaching criterion on three sentence-length responses, these responses were produced during a conversational exchange with the experimenter.

Two observational codes were used in this study. During the treatment phase each response was recorded as correct or incorrect on a trial-by-trial basis. In addition, a five-point scoring code was used to score verbal responses during sessions in which generalization to other settings and experimenters was probed. Each target response consisted of a three word sentence (e.g., "yes, I do") and was scored as follows: "one point for each correct word, and one point for each correctly ordered two-word combination" (p. 142). Only the first three words of each response were scored when longer responses were produced. Thus, a total of 5 points could be tallied for each response.

Close examination of this scoring procedure reveals that there was not a one-to-one correspondence between the numerical code and a given response. Each number in the code represented a composite score for several behaviors and it is not possible, therefore, to determine the exact nature of a response. For example, a score of 3 could represent a two-word utterance (e.g., "I do") in which the words were properly sequenced (one point for each word and one for the correct sequence) or, it could represent a response in which the three target words were produced in the wrong sequence (e.g., "Do I, yes"). Interpretive difficulties may also arise if a composite numerical code is used and interobserver agreement is obtained for the number of points assigned to verbal responses, because agreement on the numerical rating would not reflect agreement on the content of the responses. In the present example, Garcia (1974) recognized the limitations of composite scoring procedures for obtaining reliability. In addition to reporting percent agreement between the experimenter and an independent observer on the numerical ratings of verbal responses, interobserver reliability was also reported for the content of the subject's responses for this study.

As noted earlier, trial-by-trial observational codes, such as those re-viewed in the previous discussion, are among the most frequently used data collection procedures in the applied behavioral literature. It will be recalled, however, that trial-by-trial recording was only used in approximately one-third of the observational studies examined in the Kelly (1977) survey. The following sections, therefore, review data collection procedures that do not require discrete trial scoring.

Event Recording

Occasionally, experimental sessions are not subdivided into discrete trials or brief intervals and "event recording" procedures are used to monitor change in subject responding. When this data collection method is used, an observer simply records the number of responses produced by marking a data sheet with a hatch mark or a predetermined observational code or symbol. Event recording procedures appear to be most useful for studies conducted in the natural environment. Analog studies conducted under tightly controlled laboratory conditions are more likely to specify carefully the exact stimulus conditions under which responses are elicited. Alternately, naturalistic studies are generally concerned with altering behavior in settings in which the events that precede a given response are less predictable and more difficult to control. Moreover, applied investigators who conduct their research in the homes, classrooms, and so on, may wish to determine if the behavior of interest can be controlled despite extraneous variables that might naturally influence the subject's behavior. It should be noted, however, that a careful delineation of experimental conditions is necessary in both laboratory and naturalistic studies. Evaluation of experimental findings and subsequent attempts to replicate a study are dependent upon the degree of operational specificity reported.

The following example demonstrates use of "event recording" data collection procedures in a naturalistic study from the communicative disorders literature. Hart and Risley (1974) examined the effects of verbal prompts and contingent toy delivery on production of nouns, adjective-noun combinations, and compound sentences by disadvantaged children in a preschool setting. A multiple-baseline design across behaviors was used to evaluate treatment effectiveness for a group of twelve children during indoor and outdoor free play periods.

Throughout the study, data were collected by having an observer write down everything the children said during 15-minute samples of the free play activity. The recorded verbalizations were also coded on computer cards for later data analysis. Nouns, adjective-noun combinations, and compound sentences were coded separately so that the effects of treatment could be evaluated for each class of behaviors. Hart and Risley (1975, 1980) used an identical data collection procedure in their follow up study of the use and elaboration of language structures that were not specifically targeted in a previous training study.

Although issues relating to naturalistic studies are futher examined in later sections of this text, a brief consideration of the interobserver reliability data from this study seems warranted. Two types of reliability were reported by Hart and Risley (1974). First, correlation coefficients ranging from 0.83 to 0.97 were obtained for interobserver agreement on the number of nouns, adjective-noun combinations, and compound sentences produced. In addition, the level of word agreement between independent observers was 0.70. This level of agreement, somewhat below levels generally reported in laboratory settings easier to control, may reflect practical difficulties encountered in the preschool setting. It should be noted, however, that it represents a moderate degree of observer variability and this might have had a considerable impact on the accuracy of the reported data. Perhaps, observer training should be considered when moderate levels of reliability are obtained. Furthermore, it may be necessary to modify response definitions, even in naturalistic settings, if moderate levels of observer disagreement are reported.

Returning to our discussion of observational codes, it is noteworthy that several methods of data collection other than event recording are available as alternatives to trial scoring. For example, rather than simply counting behaviors as they occur during an observational period, an investigator may decide to divide the experimental session into smaller segments so that occurrence of a behavior can be monitored during specific time intervals. The two primary categories of temporal recording procedures are interval recording and time sampling.

Interval Recording and Time Sampling

The simplest of the time-based data collection procedures, interval recording, involves dividing an observational period into short intervals and having observers record the occurrence of behavior during each interval. The time of the interval is determined by the investigator and varies from one study to the next. Ten seconds appears to be a common interval, but others are also frequently employed (Kelly, 1977). Use of interval recording requires an observer to record only one occurrence or nonoccurrence of a target behavior for each observational period. Although multiple responses may occur within a given interval, a single occurrence would be recorded for that period (Kazdin, 1977b).

Time-sampling procedures are a common variation of interval recording. The investigator again divides the observation period into predetermined intervals. The observer only records the target behavior at the end of the time segment, however, and intervals of observation are followed by a specific recording period (Kelly, 1977). Responses are again scored on an occurrence / nonoccurrence basis when these procedures are used. Several variations of time-sampling data collection methods can be differentiated, depending on whether behaviors must occur throughout an entire interval to be counted as an occurrence, or just some portion of it (Powell, Martindale, and Kulp, 1975).

An example of a study that employed a time-sampling code may help to clarify the procedures used with this method of data collection. In a previously discussed study, Thompson et al. (1979) used a partial interval observational system in their examination of the effects of contingent food presentation and a lingual pushback procedure on the tongue-thrusting behavior of a cerebral palsied child. Throughout this study, the experimenters monitored the rate of occurrence of three dependent variables ("tongue out," food explusion, and chewing) to assess the efficacy of treatment. A time-sampling procedure was implemented to divide meal-time observational periods into 10–second intervals. Each interval was further divided into a 7.5–second observation segment and a 2.5–second recording segment. A cassette tape was used to designate observational and recording periods. A 10–second rest period was systematically interspersed with the observing-recording intervals.

The procedures followed in this study highlight the differences between interval recording and time-sampling procedures. In this investigation the observation periods were interrupted by carefully specified recording periods. Had interval recording been employed, the 10–second intervals would not have been subdivided and an observer could have a deleterious effect on the accuracy of the observer's recording of target behaviors. For example, if a behavior occurred during the final second of a 10–second interval, recording of that behavior could actually take place at the beginning of the subsequent interval. As a result, observation during that time would be interrupted and inaccurate and unreliable recording might occur. Although the recording periods in a time-sampling procedure might coincide with the subject's response, the investigator is likely to obtain data representative of the designated observation period.

Interval recording techniques are flexible and can be used to study discrete behaviors of any duration. It should be noted, however, that the interval selected may affect the accuracy of recorded data (Powell et al., 1975; Repp et al., 1976; Sanson-Fisher, Poole, and Dunn, 1980). Additionally, interpretive difficulties arise when this method is used because a single occurrence is usually recorded for a given interval, despite the fact that several discrete behaviors may actually occur within that interval. Similarly, when a single response is of sufficient duration to overlap scoring intervals, it will be recorded as a separate and a discrete occurrence during each consecutive interval. As a result, the number of occurrences recorded may not be an accurate indication of the true rate of frequency of behavior when interval data are utilized. It is apparent that further research is needed to develop empirical procedures for establishing appropriate recording intervals when interval and time-sampling data collection techniques are employed (Sanson-Fisher et al., 1980).

Response Duration

Investigators in communicative disorders are frequently interested in manipulating rate or frequency of occurrence of a target behavior. Occasionally, however, duration of a response may be of primary concern. For example, a response-duration code could be used for an investigator interested in lengthening the duration of a subject's esophageal phonation or reducing the pause time that precedes initiation of phonation in a severe stutterer. Unlike interval-recording procedures, this time-based method of observation does not involve subdividing an observation period into smaller recording intervals. When this procedure is used, the observer simply records the total duration of each response produced during an observation session, frequently by using a stop watch or an electronic timer. Duration measurement is most useful for recording continuous rather than discrete responses and it is, therefore, seldom used in applied communicative disorders research.

The purpose of this section has been to introduce categories of observational codes frequently used in applied behavioral research. This review is not intended to be exhaustive as there are numerous variations of the recording techniques discussed. Moreover, some methods of measurement cannot be classified in the taxonomy presented. Heward and Eachus (1979), for example, used a permanent product-recording procedure in their study of the graphic ability of hearing-impaired and aphasic children. In this study, subjects were trained to write sentences containing adjectives and adverbs, and the written responses served as the primary data.

As this example demonstrates, selection of an observational code will ultimately depend on the experimental question being investigated and the particular behavior of interest. In addition, the duration and natural frequency occurrence of that behavior, and practical considerations, such as the experience and/or cooperation of available observer-recorders, must be considered.

Once an investigator has chosen an appropriate method for gathering data, a reliable procedure must be demonstrated that accurately reflects change in subject responding. We begin to explore this issue in the following discussion.

CALCULATING INTEROBSERVER RELIABILITY

Despite the prominent role of interobserver reliability in applied research, methods of calculating interobserver agreement have only recently been examined in the literature. Ironically, the cumulative effect of this renewed interest in reliability has been to demonstrate that formulas used to derive reliability coefficients may have a marked effect on the level of agreement obtained. Furthermore, this literature has highlighted weaknesses of frequently used methods of calculation and emphasized the need to evaluate reliability coefficients in conjunction with other variables that can influence the level of agreement reported. Finally, alternate procedures have been proposed for deriving and reporting reliability data. As a result of these factors, choosing a method for calculating reliability for a given set of data is a complicated process that requires a sophisticated knowledge of the strengths and weaknesses of available alternatives. The review that follows examines developments in the literature regarding calculation and reporting of interobserver reliability. Several percentage agreement procedures will be presented, and related issues, essential for calculating or interpreting observer agreement data, are discussed.

Percentage Agreement Methods

Percentage agreement procedures have been the most recommended and widely used methods of calculating interobserver reliability in applied behavior analytic studies (Bijou et al., 1968; Hawkins and Dotson, 1975). However, the complacent attitude that seemed to prevail regarding use of such procedures has been altered by the realization that there are several pitfalls that may accompany this approach. Methods of deriving interobserver reliability using a percentage agreement approach for the total, point-to-point, occurrence and nonoccurrence methods will be examined in this section.

Total Method   Percentage agreement scores can be calculated for the total number of observations during a session, regardless of the method of data collection employed in a given study. This procedure is, however, most frequently employed when event-recording or response-duration measures are used (Kelly, 1977). Estimates of "total" reliability are obtained by dividing the smaller number recorded by an observer with the larger score recorded by a second observer. The obtained ratio is then multiplied by 100 and a percentage of agreement is obtained. For example, if two observers recorded the articulatory responses of a subject during a 100–trial treatment session, one observer might record 40 correct responses while a second observer records 50 correct responses. Using the above formula ($\frac{40}{50} \times 100$), an interjudge agreement of 80% would have been obtained.

Although total percentage methods of calculating interobserver reliability have been used in the communicative disorders literature (Jackson and Wallace, 1974), it is not an appropriate procedure, and future investigators should adopt alternative methods for calculating interjudge agreement. Total reliability methods are inadequate because they do not provide information regarding agreement on individual occurrences of behavior (Johnson and Bolstad, 1973; Hawkins and Dotson, 1975). Two observers could, for example, have perfect agreement on the total number of responses produced despite having recorded entirely different occurrences of the behavior.

Taking an extreme example, two observers might agree that 50 correct responses were produced during an experimental session in which there was a total of 100 trials. In the unlikely event that this occurred, the obtained inter-judge agreement ($\frac{50}{50} \times 100$) would be 100%. One does not know, however, the agreement for individual responses. Perhaps one observer recorded only the first fifty responses as correct, whereas the second observer recorded only the last fifty responses as correct. It is apparent that recalculation of reliability for individual occurrences of the behavior, the data of interest in single-case experimental studies, would result in total disagreement.

Although extreme, this example demonstrates the inadequacy of total percentage agreement methods of reliability calculation. More appropriate procedures will be examined in subsequent sections.

Point-to-Point Reliability   In an attempt to circumvent the inadequacies of "total" reliability procedures, many investigators obtain observer agreement on the occurrence and nonoccurrence of target behaviors on a response-by-response basis. Often referred to as *point-to-point* reliabilily, this is perhaps the most widely used method of calculating interjudge agreement in within-subject research literature (Hawkins and Dotson, 1975; Kelly, 1977). The prevalent use of point-to-point reliability procedures is, no doubt, related to the advantages it offers over alternate procedures. First, it provides an indication of the consistency and accuracy of recording for individual responses and, therefore, is closely related to the basic datum of interest in within-case experimental research (Baer, 1977a). In addition, the formula used for determining point-to-point reliability is easy to apply. Unlike correlational and other procedures frequently recommended, this method does not require a sophisticated understanding of statistics or mathematics.

To calculate point-to-point agreement, two observers independently record the behavior of a single subject according to a predetermined response definition and observational code. After the period of observation, the observers' records are examined on a response-by-response basis to determine the number of agreements and disagreements present for both occurrences and nonoccurrences (or errors) of the target response. When this approach is followed, an agreement is defined as concurrence between observers that a response did or did not occur on a given trial or during a given recording interval. Alternately, disagreements reflect instances in which one observer recorded an occurrence of an acceptable response while a second did not. After completing this analysis the following formula is used to compute the percentage of interjudge agreement:

$$\frac{\text{Total number of agreements}}{\text{Total number of agreements and disagreements}} \times 100 = \text{percentage of agreement}$$

Examination of data from a segment of a hypothetical experimental session may provide a useful demonstration of the simplicity of this method of calculation. Table 3 provides such data for two observers.

A plus (+) in the table indicates the observer recorded an occurrence of an acceptable response and a minus (−) indicates a nonoccurrence or error response. Trials for which disagreement occurred are indicated by an asterisk. It can be seen from the table that there are a total of eight agreements and two disagreements for the 10 trials presented. Using the previously presented formula ($\frac{8}{8+2} \times 100$) point-to-point interobserver reliability of 80% would be obtained.

Point-to-point interobserver reliability has considerable practical utility. As Baer (1977a) notes, "Percentage of agreement, in the interval recording (or point to point) paradigm, does have a direct and useful meaning: how often do two observers watching one subject, and equipped with the same definitions of behavior, see it occurring or not occurring at the same standard time? The . . . answers . . . are superbly useful" (pp. 117–118). Yet, despite its previously noted advantages, several important limitations to this approach are noteworthy. Hawkins and Dotson (1975), for example, demonstrate that point-to-point reliability procedures may not be sensitive to grossly inadequate response definitions or observer incompetence, and may not detect sources of bias that distort experimental findings. Thus, the accuracy of observers' recordings cannot be easily inferred from this method of calculating interobserver reliability. The basic weakness of this method relates to the fact that the agreement level obtained is a direct reflection of

Table 3. Hypothetical data depicting interobserver agreement for two observers

	Observer 1	Observer 2
Trial 1	+	+
2 *	−	+
3	+	+
4	+	+
5	+	+
6 *	+	−
7	−	−
8	−	−
9	+	+
10	+	+

Asterisks indicate disagreements.

the rate of production of the target behavior. That is, when the point-to-point method is used, and the rate of the target behavior is either very high or low, observers are certain to reach a high level of interobserver agreement (Bijou et al., 1968; Neale and Liebert, 1973; Hawkins and Dotson, 1975; Hopkins and Hermann, 1977). When extremely high rates of behavior occur during a session, agreement on these occurrences inflates point-to-point reliability. Similarly, during periods of very low rates of production of a target response, agreements on the large number of nonoccurrences inflates the obtained agreement estimate. In each of these instances, there is a high probability that agreement will be obtained on the basis of chance alone. With extreme rates of behavior a surprisingly high percentage of agreement would be expected even if observers randomly recorded their observations.

The level of chance agreement that can be expected for a given set of data is calculable if the rate of occurrence of the behavior is known. Moreover, knowledge of the probability of chance agreement is necessary for objectively evaluating percentage agreement reliability. We therefore briefly examine the formula for deriving chance agreement for point-to-point reliability measurement and present an example of this procedure. Hopkins and Hermann (1977) present the following simple formula for calculating chance agreement when overall (point-to-point) reliability is obtained:

$$\text{Chance R overall} = \frac{(0_1 \times 0_2) + (N_1 \times N_2)}{(T)^2} \times 100$$

When this formula is employed, 0_1 and 0_2 refer to the number of trials or intervals in which the first and second observer respectively record an occurrence of response. N_1 and N_2 refer to the number of trials or intervals in which the first or second observer records a nonoccurrence or error response. The total number of trials or intervals for which agreement is calculated is designated by T. Using this formula, the deleterious effects of rate or frequency of responding on reliability calculation can be demonstrated.

Suppose that independent observers recorded the frequency of correct verbal production of target sentences by an adult aphasic subject during a 100–trial experimental session. If the observers agreed that the target response was produced during only 10 of the trials, and not on 90 trials during the observed session, then the level of agreement that would be expected by chance agreement along would be:

$$\text{Chance R overall} = \frac{(10 \times 10) + (90 \times 90)}{(100)^2} \times 100 = 82\%$$

Thus, when the rate of behavior is this low, perhaps as might be expected during a baseline session, greater than 80% of the agreements obtained between independent observers would be expected on the basis of chance alone. By slightly altering this example one can also see the influence of high rates of behavior on the percentage agreement method. If the observers had recorded the behavior during a session in which they concurred the behavior had been produced during 90 trials, then the same high level of chance agreement would have been obtained. That is, overall chance agreement is:

$$\frac{(90 \times 90) + (10 \times 10)}{(100)^2} \times 100 = 82\%$$

Thus, extremely high or extremely low rates of the target behavior can spuriously inflate point-to-point reliability measurements. It appears that an estimate of the probability of chance agreement is necessary in order for interval-by-interval or point-to-point interobserver agreement to be interpretable. Reported levels of agreement must, at least, be above the level expected by chance. Methods are available for calculating whether reported levels of agreement are statistically above the level expected by chance (Hartmann, 1977; Birkimer and Brown, 1979b). However, there are presently no guidelines established for determining acceptable significance levels (Hopkins and Hermann, 1977). Although statistical approaches to reliability calculation are discussed in subsequent sections, we agree with those who reject these solutions as an undesirable departure from the behavior analytic approach to treatment research (Michael, 1974a, b; Baer, 1977a, b).

An alternative to calculating the probability of chance agreement by using the formula suggested above, is to compare obtained point-to-point reliability with a function for chance overall reliability (Hawkins and Dotson, 1975). An example of such a function provided by Hopkins and Hermann (1977) is found in Figure 26.

The graph is simple to use and provides an accurate estimate for chance reliability when observers are recording an approximately equal number of occurrences during an observation session. It should be noted that the level of overall chance agreement should be computed by using the previously presented formula when there is a difference between percentage of occurrence recorded by the observers.

As can be seen from the figure, the percentage of agreement expected by chance is presented along the ordinate, and percentage of trials or intervals in which a response occurred is presented along the abscissa. To calculate the level of overall chance reliability, one determines the point on the horizontal axis which corresponds with the percent of trials in which occurrences were recorded, and then draws a vertical line toward the function. The point on the vertical axis directly parallel to the point of intercept provides the percentage of agreement that would be expected on the basis of chance. Taking the previously presented examples, it can be seen that a vertical line drawn from either the 10% occurrence rate or the 90% point on the abscissa

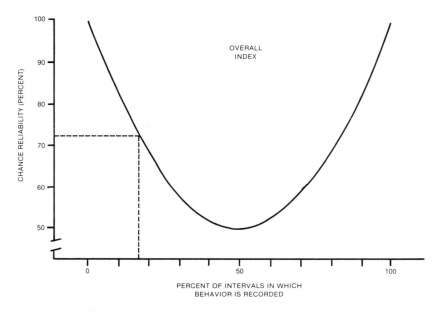

Figure 26. Overall chance reliability as a function of the percentage of intervals in which a behavior is recorded as occurring. (From Hopkins and Hermann, 1977, p. 124. Copyright by Society for the Experimental Analysis of Behavior, Inc. Reproduced by permission).

intercepts the function at approximately the 82 % point. This is in agreement with the level obtained when the formula was used to calculate the percentage of interobserver agreement expected by chance.

Although reporting chance reliability level in conjunction with point-to-point reliability calculations makes agreement coefficients more interpretable, it does not eliminate influence of rate of responding on the obtained level of agreement. Two methods of reliability calculation that attempt to circumvent the limitations of the point-to-point method by excluding inflationary effects of high and low rates of responding are discussed in the following section.

OCCURRENCE AND NONOCCURRENCE RELIABILITY

In the previous discussion of point-to-point reliability, it was noted that agreements on occurrences and nonoccurrences of a target behavior were included in calculation of the reliability coefficient. Yet, it was also noted that, depending on the rate of production of the target behavior, inclusion of agreements for either occurrences or nonoccurrences could significantly alter the level of chance agreement that could be expected. As a result of this, Bijou et al., (1968) suggested that the agreement on nonoccurrences be excluded from the reliability formula during periods of very low rates of responding and agreement on occurrences be excluded when a very high rate of responding is obtained. The reliability calculations resulting from these suggestions have been referred to as *occurrence* and *nonoccurrence* reliability, respectively. Essentially, these reliability coefficients are computed by excluding the component (occurrence or nonoccurrence) that otherwise would have an inflationary effect on obtained levels of agreement.

Like other percentage agreement methods, occurrence and nonoccurrence reliability coefficients are easy to calculate. The Hopkins and Hermann (1977) formula for computations of occurrence reliability is simply:

$$\text{Occurrence reliability} = \frac{0_{1 \text{ and } 2}}{T_0} \times 100$$

The symbol $0_{1 \text{ and } 2}$ refers to the number of trials or intervals in which two observers agree that a correct response occurred and T_0 refers to the total number of occurrence agreements and disagreements. This formula differs from the point-to-point formula presented earlier because only trials for which both observers recorded an occurrence of the target response are included as "agreements." Agreements on nonoccurrences (errors) are not considered in the computation of occurrence reliability.

Nonoccurrence reliability is the reciprocal of occurrence reliability. Essentially, interobserver agreement is computed only for trials or intervals when both observers record the nonoccurrence of a correct target behavior, and trials on which observers agree that a correct response occurred are discarded. The formula for computing nonoccurrence reliability is as follows:

$$\text{Nonoccurrence reliability} = \frac{N_{1 \text{ and } 2}}{T_n} \times 100$$

The symbol $N_{1 \text{ and } 2}$ refers to trials or intervals in which two observers agree that an acceptable response did not occur. T_n represents the total number of agreements plus disagreements for nonoccurrences.

Few examples of the use of occurrence and nonoccurrence agreement measures can be found in the applied communicative disorders literature. In fact, a review of the literature revealed only one study that had adopted these procedures (Thompson et al., 1979). We will therefore present a hypothetical example to demonstrate calculation of occurrence reliability. Before proceeding, however, it may be beneficial to review briefly a convenient method of organizing information needed to calculate these and other reliability coefficients: the 2×2 contingency table (Hartmann, 1977; Kent and Foster, 1977). Use of the contingency table may help to clarify subsequent examples, and may facilitate ease of computation for investigators wishing to apply these approaches. Contingency tables can also be used to summarize available observer agreement data and may be useful to investigators attempting to choose an observer-agreement procedure.

The data to be considered are from a hypothetical investigation of the effectiveness of a training procedure designed to teach speech-reading skills to severely hearing-impaired children. We will assume that the behavior of interest was observed during a 100-trial baseline session, and that one observer recorded 15 occurrences and 85 nonoccurrences, whereas the second observer recorded 10 occurrences and 90 nonoccurrences. Of these, interobserver agreement was reported for 10 occurrences and 80 nonoccurrences.

These data may be summarized in a 2 × 2 contingency table as shown in Figure 27. It can be seen that the "A" cell corresponds to agreements on occurrences (i.e., "$0_{1 \text{ and } 2}$"), and that the "D" cell represents agreements on nonoccurrences (i.e., "$N_{1 \text{ and } 2}$"). The remaining cells depict the disagreements recorded by the observers. Cell "B" shows the number of trials on which the first observer recorded an incorrect response and the second observer recorded a correct response. Similarly, cell "C" represents trials on which observer 1 recorded a correct response and observer 2 recorded an incorrect response. Cumulatively, cells A and D are the total number of agreements recorded, and B and C represent the total number of disagreements. Note that the sum of cells B + C provides the number of disagreements for occurrences or nonoccurrences, because there is generally no set standard for determining which observer had correctly scored a given trial. Finally, the total number of observational trials can be determined by summing all four cells (A + B + C + D).

Given the low rate of responding (number of occurrences) recorded by both observers, occurrence reliability would appear to be an appropriate

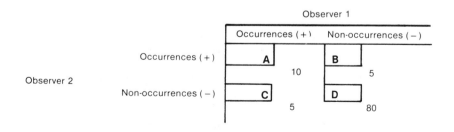

Figure 27. Data from a hypothetical investigation of the effectiveness of a training procedure designed to teach speech-reading skills to children with severe hearing impairment.

agreement statistic for these data. We will therefore compute the occurrence reliability formula for the data in the table thus:

$$\text{Occurrence reliability} = \frac{0_{1 \text{ and } 2}}{T_o} \times 100$$

$$= \frac{A}{A + B + C} \times 100$$

$$= \frac{10}{10 + 5 + 5}(100) = 50\%$$

It is apparent that this coefficient is considerably lower than currently proposed reliability guidelines of 80% or greater (Kazdin, 1977b). Proposed guidelines are, however, for point-to-point agreement only and none are available for occurrence reliability. This example is not atypical of results that might be obtained during periods of low rate of responding from an intervention study. It should be emphasized, therefore, that occurrence and nonoccurrence reliability procedures generally result in lower levels of agreement than the more frequently employed point-to-point methods, and new standards may need to be developed for what is considered an "acceptable" level of reliability when these more recent methods are used (Hawkins and Dotson, 1975). One standard proposed for evaluating occurrence and nonoccurrence methods is the use of chance agreement as a basal reliability level, the next topic of discussion.

Occurrence and nonoccurrence reliability estimates, like previously discussed point-to-point percentage agreement methods, are influenced by the rate of subject responding (Hartmann, 1977, Birkimer and Brown, 1979b). Thus, the probability of obtaining agreement on the basis of chance varies in conjunction with changes in response rate for both measures. Whereas the probability of chance level agreement increases as response rate accelerates for occurrence agreement, the reciprocal is true for the nonoccurrence method. For this method, decreases in response rate result in a higher probability of chance level agreement. The effect of rate of responding must, therefore, be considered whenever occurrence or nonoccurrence reliability is calculated or evaluated. Two procedures that deal directly with the problems created by the interrelationship between response rate and occurrence/nonoccurrence agreement levels will be considered in the following sections.

The first procedure of interest proposes that the level of agreement expected on the basis of chance should be calculated and used as a minimum standard for assessing occurrence and nonoccurrence agreement (Hawkins and Dotson, 1975). Reliability coefficients that fall below the level of agreement expected on the basis of chance alone are considered unacceptable. Hopkins and Hermann (1977) propose the following formulas for determining levels of chance agreement:

$$\text{Chance occurrence} = \frac{0_1 \times 0_2}{(T)^2} \times 100$$

$$\text{Chance nonoccurrence} = \frac{N_1 \times N_2}{(T)^2} \times 100$$

0 again refers to the number of trials for which the designated observer (subscript) recorded an occurrence of a response and N indicates the number of nonoccurrences recorded. The total number of trials compared is indicated by T. If both observers are recording approximately the same number of occurrences, Hopkins and Hermann (1977) provide the function for quickly estimating level of chance agreement for occurrence or nonoccurrence reliability in Figure 28. You will recall that the level of chance reliability is determined by first finding the point along the abscissa that represents the percentage of occurrence responses recorded for an observation session and then drawing a horizontal line until it intercepts the appropriate function. The point along the ordinate that corresponds to the place of intercept is the percentage of chance reliability.

In examining the figure it is noteworthy that the previously discussed relationship between rate of responding and chance level of agreement is clearly demonstrated. Increases in response rate above the 50% point are associated with rapidly increasing levels of chance reliability for occurrence agreement, and there is a rapid increase in the chance agreement level as the response rate falls below the 50% level for nonoccurrence reliability.

The usefulness of the chance level of agreement as a standard for assessing occurrence and nonoccurrence reliability can be demonstrated by returning to our previous example of occurrence reliability. An explicit assumption of this approach is that reliability coefficients must surpass the calculable level of chance agreement to be acceptable. We will, therefore, determine the chance level of agreement associated with the obtained 50% occurrence reliability. In our previous discussion, it was stated that the number of occurrences recorded by observer 1 was 15, whereas the second observer recorded 10 occurrences. In addition, there were 100 observational trials during the session. By employing the above formula we calculate the desired statistic as follows:

$$\text{Chance occurrence reliability} = \frac{10 \times 15}{(100)^2} \times (100) = 1.5\%$$

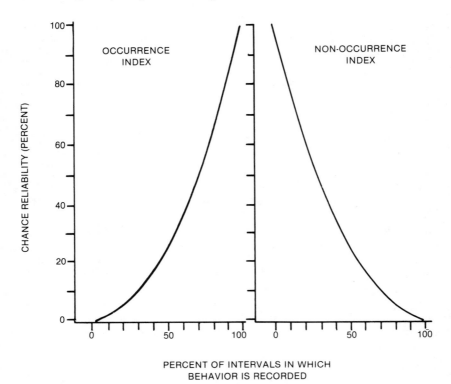

Figure 28. Occurrence and nonoccurrence chance reliability as a function of the percentage of intervals in which a behavior is recorded as occurring. (From Hopkins and Hermann, 1977, p. 124. Copyright by Society for the Experimental Analysis of Behavior, Inc. Reproduced by permission).

Given that the level of occurrence agreement expected on the basis of chance alone is less than 2%, it is evident that the obtained occurrence reliability of 50% far exceeds this level. Although the occurrence agreement is well below currently held minimum standards for point-to-point reliability, it easily surpasses the unique criteria of chance level agreement. The same conclusion is reached when the occurrence reliability function (Figure 28) is used to obtain the appropriate chance reliability level. The level of chance occurrence reliability associated with a 10% to 15% occurrence rate closely corresponds to the level determined by using the formula.

In the preceding examples occurrence reliability and chance level agreement were demonstrated, but nonoccurrence methods were not. The computation of occurrence and nonoccurrence is, however, quite similar. Moreover, the frequency of responding may be expected to change during an investigation and it has been suggested that both occurrence and non-occurrence reliability be calculated for a given study (Bijou et al., 1968; Hawkins and Dotson, 1975). As Kazdin (1977b) notes, presentation of both types of interobserver agreement would provide more useful information than either measure in isolation.

Although it is clear that measurement of occurrence and nonoccurrence reliability may be necessary to evaluate observer agreement, variations in rate of responding may make it difficult to decide when to use these procedures (Hartmann, 1977). Furthermore, it is not currently known if it would be advantageous to depict occurrence and nonoccurrence data separately or in a combined, perhaps averaged form (Hawkins and Dotson, 1975). We therefore consider an interesting means of combining these two agreement measurements into a single coefficient in the following discussion.

Combining Occurrence and Nonoccurrence Reliability

The adoption of occurrence and nonoccurrence procedures and incorporation of chance level agreement as a minimal standard of acceptance for percentage agreement methods of determining reliability may represent a considerable departure from currently prevalent assumptions of the behavior-analytic approach to intervention research. As we have seen, levels of agreement that are extremely low can be above the chance level of reliability.

Recognizing the limitations of the chance probability approach to reliability assessment, Harris and Lahey (1978) have proposed a method for combining occurrence and nonoccurrence observer agreement methods that minimizes the inflationary effects of chance agreement. Unlike the approach advocated by Hopkins and Hermann (1977), a separate determination of chance levels of agreement is not required. Instead, the proposed formula assigns weight to occurrence and nonoccurrence components of the reliability estimate according to the rate of subject responding. During periods of high rates of correct responding when agreement on occurrences is expected to inflate the reliability estimate, more weight is assigned to agreement on nonoccurrences. In effect, this diminishes the influence of chance agreement due to occurrences. Similarly, proportionately more weight is assigned to the occurrence component during periods of low rates of responding so that the inflationary effect of the large number of nonoccurrences can be minimized. Thus, the weighted formula for combining occurrence and nonoccurrence reliability compensates for the influence of chance agreement in accordance with the rate of responding.

Harris and Lahey (1978) propose the following weighted agreement (WA) formula for combining occurrence and nonoccurrence reliability.

$$WA = (0 \times U) + (N + S) \times 100$$
where
0 is the occurrence agreement score . . . ;
U is the mean proportion of unscored intervals . . . ;
N is the non-occurrence agreement score . . . ; and
S is the mean proportion of scored intervals . . .   (p. 526, 527)

The two new components in this formula that have not been discussed, the mean rates of occurrence (U) and nonoccurrence (S), function as the weighting factors. Computation of the occurrence and nonoccurrence agreement components is equivalent to the method of calculation presented in the previous sections of this chapter.

To date, no study has appeared in the communicative disorders literature that has employed the weighted agreement method of estimating interobserver reliability. We will, therefore, return to our previous example and the 2 × 2 contingency table in Figure 27 and compute "WA" using these data:

$$WA = \left(\frac{10}{10 + 5 + 5} \quad \frac{0.85 + 0.90}{2} \right) + \left(\frac{80}{80 + 5 + 5} \quad \frac{0.15 + 0.10}{2} \right) \times 100 \quad (1)$$

$$= \left((0.50) \quad (0.88) \right) \quad + \quad \left((.89) \quad (0.13) \right) \times 100 \quad (2)$$

$$= \left((0.44) \quad + \quad (0.12) \right) \times 100 \quad (3)$$

$$= 56\% \quad (4)$$

In general, it can be seen that the 56% WA is similar to the occurrence reliability of (50%) reported for the same data. Examination of line 2 of computation reveals the reason for this. Nearly 90% (0.88) of the weighting in the example is associated with the occurrence score and approximately 13% (0.13) with the nonoccurrence score. Similar results would be expected between the nonoccurrence reliability score and the weighted agreement score, had the example been selected from a period of high rate of responding. When extremely high or low rates of behavior are produced during an observational period, differences between the weighted agreement score and the appropriate occurrence or nonoccurrence index will be negligible.

Harris and Lahey (1978) discuss several potential advantages of using the weighted agreement formula. They note that it is similar to currently used point-to-point measures because a single percentage agreement score is obtained within the 0% to 100% range. In addition, the formula compensates for the influence of rate of responding and chance level of agreement and combines occurrence and nonoccurrence reliability scores. It is suggested that a standard of, perhaps, 80% or better could be adopted to assess weighted agreement scores. Finally, WA is purportedly most useful when considerable variability is apparent in the response rate of target behaviors.

To this point in our discussion we have emphasized percentage agreement methods of calculating observer agreement and reviewed various methods of compensating for the inflationary effects that rate of subject responding may have on these measurements. In the following section, the discussion is extended by including a brief consideration of alternatives to the percentage agreement approach.

Graphic Approaches to Interobserver Agreement

Hawkins and Dotson (1975) were among the first authors to suggest that observer-recorded data should be graphically displayed so that interobserver reliability data would be available for direct inspection. They noted that when both types of data are displayed, the research consumer can examine whether one of the observers tended to over- or underestimate experimental effects. Bias might, for example, be indicated if the primary observer consistently recorded lower rates of behavior during sessions in which reliability is assessed as compared with other sessions. The graphic approach to reliability assessment may, therefore, provide a useful alternative to the percentage agreement methods.

Birkimer and Brown (1979a) have presented a graphic approach that summarizes obtained and chance reliability data. They recommend that each observer's percentage of disagreements $\left(\frac{\text{Number of disagreements}}{\text{Total number of trials}} \right) \times 100$ be plotted on the same graph as the primary experimental data for everyday reliability is assessed. This percentage of disagreement may be graphed as a vertical band centered around the mean rate of target behavior recorded by the two observers. The upper and lower limits of the range are bounded by the two observers' response rates. This disagreement band then represents the range of observer disagreements for the occurrence of the target behavior. The area beneath the lower limit of the disagreement range represents percentage of observer agreement for the occurrences of the target behavior, and the area above the range represents the percentage of observer agreements for nonoccurrences of the target behavior. Thus, by calculating a single reliability index for percentage of disagreements and plotting it along with the rates of occurrence reported, all of the information needed to determine point-to-point, occurrence, and nonoccurrence reliability is provided.

Birkimer and Brown (1979a) also advocate calculating the level of chance disagreement

$$\frac{(0_1 \times N_2) + (N_1 \times 0_2)}{T_2} \times 100$$

and graphing it around the mean of the two observers' response rates. The chance disagreement level would be graphically displayed within the vertical chance disagreement range while the area below the chance disagreement range would provide the chance occurrence reliability and the area above the range the chance level of agreement on nonoccurrences. These data provide the information needed to assess whether the obtained reliability exceeds the minimal standard of the calculated chance level. Birkimer and Brown (1979a) summarized their graphic approach presented in Figure 29.

Birkimer and Brown's (1979a) reliability suggestions have been throughly discussed in invited commentaries presented in conjunction with the original publication, and interested readers are referred to these reviews for additional information. Furthermore, a succinct summary of this approach is available (Hopkins, 1979).

The graphic approach to interobserver reliability is relatively easy to employ, comprehensive, and provides a direct visual display of reliability data. Moreover, it may be useful for detecting bias in observer recordings and evaluating the believability of experimental findings (Hawkins and Dotson,

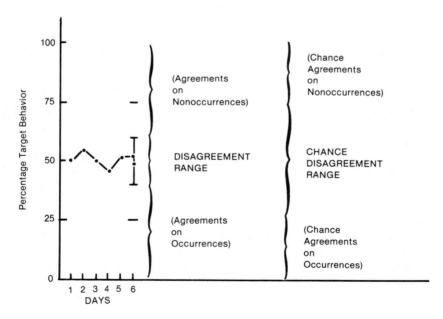

Figure 29. Use of disagreement range to partition all observation occasions into those producing agreements on occurrences, disagreements and agreements on nonoccurrences, and use of chance disagreement range to show chance rates of agreements on occurrences, disagreements, and agreements on nonoccurrences. (From Birkimer and Brown, 1974, p. 528. Copyright by Society for the Experimental Analysis of Behavior, Inc. Reproduced by permission).

1975; Birkimer and Brown, 1979a). However, several limitations of this method of reliability assessment have been identified. Kratochwill and Wetzel (1977), for example, note that the major benefits of this approach occur before publication. That is, if graphic display of reliability data reveals that only one of two observers consistently records an experimental effect, obtained results are unreliable and further refinement of the study protocol is needed. These authors also note that additional graphing necessitated by this approach would be expensive and further complicate the task of assessing experimental results through visual inspection. This latter point appears to be the most critical, because visual analysis of applied behavioral data is a difficult task (DeProspero and Cohen, 1979), and addition of reliability observers' data would be expected to add to the complexity of the evaluative process.

The graphic presentation of reliability data can be viewed as an extension of the percentage and chance agreement methods. In addition to a visual display of observer data, the graphic approach extends these methods by providing a convenient means of determining point-to-point, occurrence/nonoccurrence agreement and their associated levels of chance with a minimum of calculation. Moreover, the percentage-agreement, chance-agreement, and graphic approaches are in keeping with the applied behavioral tradition of relying on data that directly represent the behavior of interest.

Statistical Approaches to Interobserver Reliability

Statistical approaches to interobserver reliability assessment have been used infrequently in applied behavior literature (Kelly, 1977). However, increased recognition of the limitations of the percentage agreement methods has prompted a renewed interest in application of statistical procedures to this facet of within-subject experimental designs. We therefore briefly consider statistical methods of reliability measurement.

Perhaps the most frequently employed statistic used to assess interobserver agreement is the Pearson product-moment correlation (r). This statistic provides an indication of the degree of linear association between the data reported by two observers for sessions in which reliability is evaluated. The association between the observer data is generally reported as occurring within a range of 0.0 to 1.0 and fractions that approximate 1.0 indicate a stronger relationship between sets of data. In addition to the Pearson r, the correlation statistics of phi (θ) and Kappa (K) have been recently discussed in the literature (Hartmann, 1977).

Limitations of the correlational approach to reliability assessment are well known (Kazdin, 1977b; Neale and Liebert, 1973). Correlation coefficients do not indicate trial-by-trial level of agreement, and they are, therefore, similar to the "total" percentage agreement approach. That is, a high coefficient may be obtained despite the fact that observers seldom agreed on the scoring of individual responses. In addition, a high correlation coefficient will be obtained even though a large disagreement range is evident if the disagreement range is relatively stable across observation sessions.

In addition to correlation statistics, several authors have recently suggested using probability theory as a basis for evaluating reliability (Yelton, Wildman, and Erickson, 1977; Birkimer and Brown, 1979b). Like previously discussed reliability approaches, these methods attempt to determine whether obtained agreement levels might be expected on the basis of chance alone. Birkimer and Brown (1979b), for example, have suggested a "50–10–10 (90) rule" for assessing reliability. They note that for 50 or more observations, when the disagreement level is less than or equal to 10% and the rate of responding is between 10% and 90%, it is highly unlikely that the agreement rate is a result of chance $(P \leq 0.01)$. Stated otherwise, on the average, there is only one chance in 100 that a reliability rate calculated under these circumstances is the result of chance agreement.

A major limitation of these and other statistical procedures used to assess reliability stems from the fact that valuable information is lost in the calculation (Kratochwill and Wetzel, 1977). In addition, statistical coefficients do not directly represent the level of observer agreement. As previously noted, a correlation coefficient of, for example, 0.70 does not mean that the observers agreed on the scoring of 70% of the experimental trials. Furthermore, statistical approaches in general are often far removed from the data of interest, the subject's behavior. As a result, there is a possibility that investigators may "lose touch" with their data (Michael, 1974a, b). Finally, the philosophy of using statistics may be seen as contrary to the basic tenets of the applied-behavior analytic approach (Baer, 1977b). Although such procedures may reveal statistically significant differences, these differences may not be of a sufficient magnitude to be clinically meaningful and, as a result, clinically weak variables may be uncovered and studied. This is in opposition to the applied behavioral belief that investigations should be restricted to variables expected to be clinically powerful and socially significant.

ADDITIONAL CONSIDERATIONS

In reviewing the reliability procedures it is important to remind ourselves that few guidelines are available for choosing among the alternative methods. The ultimate choice of a procedure will be influenced by the rate and variability of the subject's response, as well as practical exigencies such as the investigator's willingness to use relatively new and unfamiliar approaches to reliability assessment. It must be admitted, however, that there is little empirical data to assist investigators in the decision-making process. Cone (1979) underscored this point when he stated, "Unfortunately, appreciation of the potential value of...the 'I've got a better agreement measure' literature must be based solely on the authors' skill at rational appeal...It seems odd that the requirement of demonstrated control of meaningful behavior has not been applied to papers dealing with agreement measures'' (p. 571). The state of the art in reliability assessment in applied studies puts the investigator in the uncomfortable position of having to select among methodological options which are, for the most part, intuitively attractive but untested.

Despite the limited amount of data available, selection of a reliability estimate is not an arbitrary process. Baer (1977a) offers the following comments on the selection process: "For applied behavior analysis, choice among estimates can be guided by (1) the avoidance of allowing the reliability of occurrence from influencing the reliability of non-occurrence, and vice-versa; and (2) by the apparent, face meaning of the estimate's calculation technique" (p. 117). Regarding the first suggestion, we have seen that inclusion of agreements on occurrences has an inflationary effect on reliability coefficients during periods of high rates of correct responding, and inclusion of nonoccurrence agreements has an inflationary effect during periods of low rates of responding. There is, in effect, a high level of chance agreement that can be expected during high or low rates of responding whenever point-to-point agreement procedures are utilized. The following guidelines are therefore suggested to counteract the effect of rate of responding on interobserver agreement. First, point-to-point agreement procedures should not be used in isolation. Unless the rate of responding is approximately 50%, point-to-point measures are highly influenced by rate of responding. Therefore the level of chance agreement should be calculated and reported whenever a percentage agreement estimate is utilized (Hawkins and Dotson, 1975; Hopkins and Hermann, 1977). Reliability levels that fall below the chance level agreement do not meet minimal standards of acceptability. During periods of low rates of responding, perhaps 50% or less, point-to-point and occurrence reliability data, and their respective levels of chance agreements, should be calculated. The point-to-point methods are familiar to most investigators and, therefore, would provide a helpful yardstick for evaluating agreement data. In addition, occurrence data would provide a measure of reliability not influenced by the biasing effects of the nonoccurrence agreements included in the calculation of the point-to-point measure. Likewise, during periods of very low rates of responding when the occurrence reliability coefficient might be highly influenced by a single occurrence disagreement (Hawkins and Dotson, 1975), the point-to-point data would provide a more stable estimate of agreement.

Just as the simultaneous use of occurrence reliability complements point-to-point measures during low rates of responding, nonoccurrence measures are particularly beneficial when rate of responding exceeds 50%. The familiar point-to-point estimate and the less biased and more variable nonoccurrence measure, when evaluated against their calculable levels of chance agreement, provide a balanced means of assessing observer-agreement data. If the point-to-point and nonoccurrence coefficients are comfortably above their respective chance levels, an important minimal criteria for accepting the data has been achieved.

In the preceding discussion of percentage agreement methods, we have not considered the role of the weighted average (combined) method (Harris and Lahey, 1978) of reliability calculation. As we have previously noted, the coefficient derived from this approach approximates the level of agreement obtained by using the nonoccurrence or occurrence formulas during periods of very high or low rates of responding closely. Thus, at extreme rates of responding when a procedure is needed to complement point-to-point estimates, the WA formula does not appear to offer additional benefits over those provided by the occurrence/nonoccurrence formulas. Moreover, the combined approach generally results in a lower level of agreement than would be obtained using the point-to-point method, and guidelines for evaulating this more conservative estimate are not currently available. Although this is also true of occurrence and nonoccurrence estimates, these methods can easily be used in conjunction with the more familiar point-to-point approach. The weighted average approach is much more likely to be used in isolation and, may therefore be difficult to interpret. Finally, although Harris and Lahey (1978) contend that the combined approach may be most useful during periods of high variability, it is not clear that any additional benefit is gained from using this method over the recommended procedure of presenting point-to-point, occurrence or nonoccurrence, and chance level data.

Two general categories of reliability calculation, graphic and statistical approaches, should be considered before closing this discussion. The graphic method proposed by Birkimer and Brown (1979a) is basically an extension of the procedures we have recommended. All of the data necessary to determine the obtained and chance percentage agreements for point-to-point, occurrence, and nonoccurrence reliability are available when this approach is employed. We do not agree, however, that the advantages of this approach, which have previously been discussed, outweigh the major problems it presents by complicating the visual inspection of data. Finally, our reasons for rejecting the statistical approach have been previously outlined and are elaborated on in another chapter of this text.

This review has favored the chance level and percentage agreement method for evaluating observer agreement data. It must be emphasized, however, that the chance level criterion suggested is only one of several important considerations that must be weighed before determining the acceptability of an agreement coefficient. The obtained reliability must, for example, meet the consumer's standard for a minimally acceptable agreement level. Kazdin (1977a, b) has indicated that the 80% agreement level is often considered a minimal level acceptable for point-to-point agreement. The absolute value accepted may vary depending on the nature of the study, types of subjects, and the observational code employed. Generally accepted standards for occurrence/nonoccurrence reliability have yet to be established. In addition to the chance criterion and the minimally established level of acceptable interobserver agreement, other factors, such as the possible sources of bias that may confound estimates, must be considered when assessing reliability. These factors will be discussed in the next and final section of this chapter.

INTEROBSERVER RELIABILITY, ACCURACY, AND BIAS

The purpose of assessing interobserver reliability is to evaluate the accuracy of behavioral observations (Hawkins and Dotson, 1975). It is not surprising therefore, that many investigators assume that reliable observations are synonymous with accurate observations. Ironically, this is an incorrect assumption because levels of interobserver agreement are not good predictors of the objectivity of behavioral recordings. It is important, therefore, to distinguish between interobserver agreement and accuracy of the recordings from which levels of agreement are determined. Unfortunately, accuracy of behavioral recordings cannot be assured even when target behaviors are carefully defined, recorded with an appropriate observational code, and calculated with a procedure that compensates for the inflationary effects rate of responding may have on a reliability estimate. Several subtle forms of bias may adversely affect the level of interobserver agreement reported. The following hypothetical example highlights the distinction between reliability and accuracy and demonstrates how the accuracy of data can be unknowingly compromised.

One of the factors that may contribute to reduced intelligibility of children with severe hearing loss is excessive hypernasality (Nober, 1967; Ling, 1976). One might, therefore, design a study to investigate the effectiveness of training procedures to decrease the amount of hypernasality produced by hearing-impaired individuals. In an attempt to satisfy the need for observer reliability in such a study, the experimenter and an observer might judge the subject's responses on a nasality rating scale. In addition, the reliability judge might be present at some of the sessions in each phase of the experiment; and after the sessions in which interjudge agreement was obtained, the observer's recordings could be compared with the experimenter's and percentage of agreement could be computed.

If a high level of interobserver agreement was obtained on the nasality ratings, and the agreed-upon scores reflected a clinically significant reduction in hypernasality, the investigators might conclude that treatment had been effective. As previously noted, however, acceptable levels of reliability are necessary but not sufficient to insure accurate observations. Let us briefly consider several factors that might have affected the accuracy of the observer ratings without influencing the obtained level of agreement. Single-case experimental designs are frequently conducted in applied settings and often the treatment being investigated is one with which the experimenters have had previous clinical experience. Suppose, therefore, that the observer and the experimenter in the hypothetical example have both used the training procedures that were being investigated and both believed them to be efficacious. The opportunity for inaccurate recordings would be present in the situation simply because the observers expected to witness a predicted outcome. Bias due to expectancy may be particularly powerful when combined with feedback contingent on the independent observer's performance (O'Leary, Kent, and Kanowitz, 1975). This additional factor might have been present in our example if the experimenter and the observer had been co-workers and had discussed their perception of the subject's performance and any discrepancies apparent in their ratings. Moreover, given the communication between the co-workers, an additional source of bias may have entered into the hypothetical study. That is, the observers' adherence to operational definitions of hypernasality might have changed or drifted in the same direction as the study progressed. If this occurred, close agreement could have been obtained between the observers even though they were not scoring the behavior according to predetermined observational definitions. Studies have, in fact, demonstrated that "observer drift" can occur in applied studies that rely on human observers as the primary method of data collection (Kent et al., 1974, 1977). Another source of bias that may have been present in our hypothetical example relates to the fact that the observer was present during selected sessions of each experimental phase of the study. This in itself may have set up situations in which bias could occur. As Harris and Ciminero (1978) have demonstrated, witnessing application of experimental contingencies during treatment phases influences observer behavior. Thus, the independent observer's scoring may actually reflect the pattern of consequation rather than the accuracy of responding.

Although the above example demonstrates several sources of bias that may occur in applied research, this does not exhaust the confounds discussed in the literature. For example, it has been demonstrated that an observer's awareness that the reliability of his recordings is being monitored may also affect the accuracy of the observations (Reid, 1970; Romanczyk et al., 1973; and Kent, et al., 1977). Reid (1970), for example, demonstrated differences of 25% between the level of agreement obtained when observers were aware that they were being monitored versus the level achieved when covert reliability checks were made. Thus, observer "reactivity" to awareness that the accuracy of his or her recording is being assessed may, in itself, have a marked effect on the level of agreement reported.

Factors such as observer expectancy and feedback, observer drift, witnessing of consequation, and reactivity should be considered and minimized when designing reliability procedures for an applied investigation. Several reviews that have considered these and other sources of bias in reliability assessment provide more detailed discussions of these topics (Kazdin, 1977a, b; Kent and Foster, 1977). These summaries also detail suggestions for controlling sources of bias that may affect reliability estimates. Investigators should, for example, attempt to minimize the effects of observer expectancy and feedback by minimizing feedback provided regarding the accuracy of the observers' recordings. Similarly, leading observers to believe that they will be covertly monitored throughout an investigation may reduce the deleterious effects of observer reactivity and enhance the accuracy of recording. The actual use of unobtrusive reliability checks may also be considered (Kazdin, 1979). This would minimize any feedback that might be obtained from nonverbal cues of the reliability observer and make it more difficult for the primary observer to discriminate between sessions in which agreement levels are checked. Evidence suggests that observations from video recordings or via a one-way mirror may result in agreement levels comparable to *in vivo* observations (Kent et al., 1974). Availability of video recording equipment can provide another means of controlling bias during reliability assessment. Reliability obtained from randomly presented taped segments of various phases of an experiment may reduce the level of bias by reducing expectations based on the observer's previous knowledge of the subject's contingency history. Finally, the use of several reliability observers throughout the course of an investigation may provide a means of determining whether these observers who have recorded a significant portion of a study have drifted from response definitions. Occasionally retraining observers to a criterion level on standard examples of behavior may help to ensure accuracy of observational data.

SCHEDULING RELIABILITY SESSIONS

It would appear that the disciplines within the area of communicative disorders may be particularly susceptible to sources of bias that may affect reliability because of their reliance on perceptual judgments as a standard for accuracy. It is important, therefore, that the above suggestions be incorporated into applied intervention studies of communicative impairments whenever possible. A final precaution that might also be considered concerns scheduling of reliability sessions. As with other aspects of experimental design, the specific number or frequency of reliability checks cannot be dictated. However, it would appear that investigators should be sensitive to the need for frequent assessment of interobserver agreement. At a minimum, reliability should be probed in every experimental phase and during each session in which training criterion is reached. The exact number of checks conducted will vary, depending on the particular factors involved in an investigation. Ideally, a second observer should score each experimental session in conjunction with the primary observer. Unfortunately, applied investigators have fallen woefully short of this ideal. In a survey of data collection procedures published in the *Journal of Applied Behavior Analysis* during a 7–year period, Kelly (1977) reported that only 9% of the relevant studies obtained reliability checks in each session. Perhaps even more surprising, a meager 23% of the studies surveyed conducted reliability checks during each experimental condition. It would appear from these data that our suggestions for minimal frequency of reliability assessment are not currently being met. It is hoped that the renewed interest in reliability procedures evident in the literature will result in an increased appreciation for the importance of interobserver reliability and an associated increase in the number of reliability sessions routinely conducted in applied behavioral studies.

SUMMARY

The importance of the reliability of observer-recorded data has been overlooked in the applied literature and problems relating to observational recording procedures have been given little consideration in the area of communicative disorders. Therefore, the purpose of this chapter has been to present an in-depth discussion of interobserver reliability and observational coding methods and to relate this information to applied communicative disorders research. We begin our discussion with a consideration of operational definitions and direct measurement techniques, two factors that directly affect reliability. After this, a review of observational codes commonly employed in within-subject investigations was presented and examples were provided to demonstrate when each coding procedure is most applicable. Electromechanical, trial-by-trial, event-recording, interval-recording, and response-duration measurement techniques were considered.

Methods of calculating interobserver reliability were assessed in the second half of this chapter. Percentage agreement methods were emphasized throughout the discussion, and total, point-to-point, occurrence, nonoccurrence, and weighted-agreement approaches were considered. Graphic and statistical methods for calculating interobserver reliability were also briefly discussed. Several advantages and limitations were presented for each of the procedures reviewed, and the adverse effect of high and low rates of responding on the level of reliability was discussed. It was concluded that percentage-agreement methods should be used in conjunction with procedures for calculating the level of chance agreement associated with extreme rates of responding. The chapter concluded with a discussion of subtle confounds and scheduling problems that may interfere with reliability assessment.

Beyond the Basic Designs

6

Several within-subject designs are available for addressing issues concerned with comparing the effectiveness of more than one treatment. Discrepancies are found in the names applied to the designs and how they function (Barlow and Hayes, 1979; Ulman and Sulzer-Azaroff, 1975; Kazdin and Hartmann, 1978; Hersen and Barlow, 1976; Kratochwill and Levin, 1980). The designs have some features in common, however, regardless of how they are labeled, placing them in the same purpose category. In this section, the design encompassing the most components for comparing treatments will be described. It is called the *alternating-treatments design* by Barlow and Hayes (1979), and labeled differently by other authors. We are treating these as modifications of the alternating-treatments design and describe them briefly. Also included in this chapter are descriptions and designs that allow more thorough evaluations of treatment components or other events in treatment programs. They consist of the *interaction design, changing criterion design,* and the *multiple-probe design.* The chapter ends with consideration of procedures for probing generalization.

ALTERNATING-TREATMENTS DESIGN

The function of the alternating-treatments design (ATD) is a comparison of two or more conditions. The purpose is to determine which condition is more effective for changing one behavior. The number of treatments evaluated may vary. It is possible to compare treatment with no-treatment as well as comparing two or more treatments. The treatments or conditions are administered simultaneously or concurrently in that they occur during the same phase, in fact, usually each condition is presented each day during the experimental phase. The treatments are alternated rapidly and counterbalancing is required.

Counterbalancing controls for order affects of one treatment always following the other, and for extraneous variables that might affect the behavior as much or more than the treatments. The variables may include time of day each treatment is administered, the experimenters providing treatment, or settings if treatment is administered by more than one experimenter at different time periods and settings. For example, if treatment 1 were always administered in the morning and treatment 2 in the afternoon, it would be difficult to isolate the effect of the treatment from the time of day it was administered. Similarly, if one experimenter always administered treatment 1 and another treatment 2, it is possible that the more effective treatment was successful because of the characteristics of the experimenter administering it. By shifting time periods, experimenters, and settings across training sessions, it is possible to rule out the influence of these extraneous variables. Counterbalancing of treatments, experimenters, time periods, and settings is used for control purposes. If several variables are to be accounted for, the balancing follows the method used to form Latin squares. An example of a design for counterbalancing two treatments offered in two different time periods by one experimenter in one setting is presented in Table 4.

Through alternating and counterbalancing treatments, the effect of the particular time period is controlled, and so are sequencing effects. Alternation is randomized in the above example in order to prevent a pattern for treatment presentations from developing; however, the alternating-treatments design demands that the treatments be administered an equal number of times. In the table, notice that both treatments are presented a total of eight times, four in the morning and four in the afternoon, although the same sequence is not repeated across the eight sessions. The study is balanced for treatment order and for morning and afternoon influences.

The example in Table 4 is less complex than customary in applied research. Frequently, more than one experimenter administers the treatments. If so, three variables need to be counterbalanced: treatment order, time of administration, and the individuals administering treatment. It is necessary to demonstrate that a particular treatment is effective regardless of when it is offered or who administers it. To control for both variables the design would conform to the form presented in Table 5. Clearly the design is counterbalanced for all possible permutations of the variables so that each experimenter administers each treatment in both time periods during the course of the study. Five days would be insufficient, however, to complete

Table 4. Design for comparing two treatments administered at different time periods

Time Period				Days				
	1	2	3	4	5	6	7	8
A.M.	Tr_1[a]	Tr_2	Tr_2	Tr_1	Tr_2	Tr_2	Tr_1	Tr_1
P.M.	Tr_2	Tr_1	Tr_1	Tr_2	Tr_1	Tr_1	Tr_2	Tr_2

[a] Tr_1, Treatment 1; Tr_2, Treatment 2.

Table 5. Design for evaluating two treatments administered by two experimenters at two different time periods

Time	Days					
	1	2	3	4	5	n
A.M.	$T_1, E_1{}^a$	T_1, E_2	T_2, E_1	T_2, E_2	—	
P.M.	T_2, E_2	T_2, E_1	T_1, E_2	T_1, E_1	—	

$^a T_1$, Treatment 1; T_2, treatment 2; E_1, experimenter 1; E_2, experimenter 2.

the study. Repetitions of the various permutations would be essential before the influence of extraneous variables could be ruled out.

It is possible to vary other features during the study. For instance, the treatments can be administered in more than one setting. When the setting is varied, the design must account for the different locations. Agents, times of day, and settings constitute the "stimulus conditions" to be accounted for by counterbalancing (Kazdin and Hartmann, 1978).

As mentioned, comparisons in the alternating-treatments design may vary. In comparing a treatment with a no-treatment condition, treatment would be alternated with no-treatment and the no-treatment condition constitutes an extended baseline. Or, two or more treatments can be compared. Browning and Stover (1971), labeling their design the *simultaneous-treatment design*, illustrate the components in the following manner:

$$
A \text{———} \underset{D}{\overset{B}{C}} \text{———} B \text{ or } C \text{ or } D
$$

In the drawing, A stands for baseline, the vertically lined $B - C - D$ represent three different interventions to be compared concurrently, and the final B or C or D indicates that in the last phase of the study the treatment found most effective during the experimental phase is applied. That is, the same treatment is now administered by all experimenters in all settings and time periods to determine if the behavior continues to change in the appropriate direction when the most effective treatment is administered.

Investigators should keep in mind that the more treatments tested, and the more variables present in the stimulus condition, the more complex the design becomes. Each treatment must be counterbalanced and so do all the extraneous variables. Kazdin and Hartmann (1978), who discuss simultaneous-treatment designs, suggest that no more than two or three treatments be compared in one study. Otherwise, the design becomes too cumbersome.

A component emphasized by investigators is association of each condition with a discriminative stimulus (Barlow and Hayes, 1979; Ulman and

Sulzer-Azaroff, 1975). The stimulus indicates which treatment is to be administered. Not all proponents of the design are equally adamant on this point (Kazdin and Hartmann, 1978). The reason for the discriminative stimulus is to allow the subject to differentiate the treatments from each other; to identify which treatment is in effect. The argument is that if discriminative stimuli are not used and the treatments have no differential effects, it would not be possible to ascertain whether the treatments were equally effective or ineffective, or if the subject was just unable to distinguish between them. Why the subject has to make that distinction is unclear. Possibly, discriminative stimuli would be more useful in studies comparing treatments that differ very little from each other, but unnecessary when treatments are clearly different. At any rate, using different stimuli supposedly facilitates the subject's discrimination of treatments, which in turn saves time during the experimental phase. The point is that if distinctive stimuli are not introduced, more sessions will be required before the subject is aware that different treatments are being administered.

The discriminative stimuli could be different experimenters or different settings, each associated with one of the treatments, or for that matter, any of the variables in the "stimulus conditions" in which the experiment is conducted. Use of these variables poses problems, however, for these are the very conditions to be rapidly alternated and counterbalanced. Because of this, they would prevent formation of a discrimination. To circumvent the problem, alternations are sometimes programmed to occur less frequently than required by the design. Another way to avoid the problem is to institute the counterbalancing only after the discrimination has already been formed by the subject. Otherwise, rapid alternations and counterbalancing at the beginning of the experimental phase may well prevent formation of a discrimination by the subject.

Not all discriminative stimuli must be counterbalanced. Neither do all studies employ supplementary discriminative stimuli, relying instead on the notion that the treatments are sufficiently distinctive to allow discrimination between them.

Stimuli that do not require counterbalancing include events apart from the stimuli composing the treatment complex, although once employed they may be viewed as part of the treatment conditions. For example, differently colored lights designating different treatments could be considered peripheral stimuli. This is not to say that they could not form confounding variables; but this is an unlikely prospect, because they are further removed from the procedures than are, for example, experimenters or treatment periods.

Lately, instructions have been introduced as discriminative stimuli in alternating-treatments design studies. The completeness of instructions varies across studies from simple statements, such as "This is treatment A" or "This is treatment B," to detailed explanations of the treatment procedure. Inasmuch as studies have demonstrated that behavioral changes can be obtained with instructions alone, their use in alternating-treatments studies must be considered in evaluating intervention effectiveness. Instructions become procedural components; they are included in conclusions regarding the effectiveness of an intervention procedure.

Need for establishing discriminative stimuli is determined by the investigator and may be related to whether the treatments differ quantitatively or qualitatively, or how much they differ. For example, if treatment 1 consists of a 1–minute period of music for fluency and treatment 2 of a 2–minute period of music for the same behavior, the subject might require a long time to distinguish treatments because they differ quantitatively and the difference is small. Instructions specifying which music period is in effect could facilitate differentiation. On the other hand, if one treatment consists of imitation and another of minimal verbal cues for word training, the subject might have less difficulty distinguishing quickly between the two treatments because they differ on many dimensions. When discriminative stimuli are used, they need to be appropriate to the behaviors studied. A few of the stimuli used in studies have included printed signs specifying the treatment in effect (Ulman and Sulzer-Azaroff, 1975), light off or on to cue which condition is in effect (Murphy, Doughty, and Nunes, 1979) and differently colored cards each associated with one treatment (Kazdin and Geesey, 1977). The number of alternating-treatments design studies is small, and use of discriminative stimuli infrequent, although they appear to be on the increase.

The number of phases in an alternating-treatments design study varies, but three are proposed: a baseline phase, the experimental-treatments phase, and a phase in which the most effective treatment from the experimental phase is administered. Although the treatments are alternated and conditions counterbalanced, results usually are not presented graphically to reflect them. A hypothetical design is shown in Table 6, and results from the hypothetical study in Figure 30.

In Table 6 on the first baseline day, experimenter 1 (E_1) measures the behavior, the dependent variable in the morning, whereas experimenter 2 (E_2) measures the behavior in the afternoon. On day 2 the experimenters reverse time periods and again on days 3 and 4 of baseline. Alternating experimenters in the two time periods allows observation of behavioral changes as a function of the person measuring the behavior and the time at which it is measured before introduction of treatment.

On the fifth day, if stability criterion is met in baseline, the two interventions (I_1, I_2) are initiated in the experimental phase. Time periods, interventions, and experimenters are alternated and counterbalanced over 8 days

Table 6. Design for two treatments administered by two experimenters at two different time periods

Time	Baseline				Experimental phase								Application phase	
	Days													
	1	2	3	4	5	6	7	8	9	10	11	12	13	14
A.M.	$E_1-I_0^a$	E_2-I_0	E_1-I_0	E_2-I_0	E_1-I_1	E_1-I_2	E_2-I_1	E_2-I_2	E_1-I_1	E_1-I_2	E_2-I_1	E_2-I_2	$E_{1-2}-I_E$	$E_{1-2}-I_E$
P.M.	E_2-I_0	E_1-I_0	E_2-I_0	E_1-I_0	E_2-I_2	E_2-I_1	E_1-I_2	E_1-I_1	E_2-I_2	E_2-I_1	E_1-I_2	E_1-I_1	$E_{1-2}-I_E$	$E_{1-2}-I_E$

$^a E_1$, Experimenter 1; E_2, experimenter 2; I_0, no intervention; I_1, intervention 1; I_2, intervention 2; I_E, most effective intervention.

of treatment. Each combination or permutation of time, experimenter, and intervention is repeated once. For example, the combination E_1-I_2 in the morning and E_2-I_1 in the afternoon is designated to occur twice during the experiment. The number of repetitions is determined by experimental requirements; however, one repetition is a minimum number. Further, if stability is not attained with the number planned, repetitions are increased.

In the final phase the experimenters and time periods are neither alternated nor counterbalanced. Instead, both experimenters administer the most effective treatment from the experimental phase in the morning and afternoon sessions. The number of days in this phase is decided arbitrarily. Primarily, the investigator wishes to demonstrate performance maintenance, or even improvement, from the experimental phase. Two or three days may be reasonable unless the investigator wishes an even more convincing demonstration by extending the phase.

Hypothetical results from the hypothetical study are presented in Figure 30. Neither the experimenters nor the time of day affected the rate of occurrence of the behavior. Baseline data show a low rate regardless of the measurement situation. Baseline provides evidence that experimenters and time periods will not confound results. Stability of the response allows introduction of treatments on day 5 as planned.

Comparison of the effectiveness of the two treatments (T_1, T_2) in the experimental phase reveals that behavior changed each time either treatment

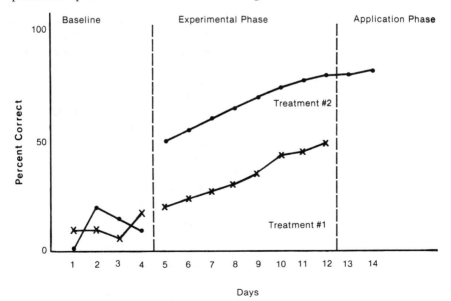

Figure 30. Hypothetical data in the three phases of an alternating treatments design.

was administered, but the behavior changed more with treatment 2. Each day, the behavior increased more in the session in which treatment 2 was in effect, regardless of whether E_1 or E_2 administered treatment in the morning or afternoon. The clear separation of data points across treatment days attests to the superiority of treatment 2.

Effectiveness of treatment 2 continues to be demonstrated in the final phase of the study. Behavior increased slightly and was maintained at 80% occurrence on the two final days of the experiment when only treatment 2 was administered.

A word of caution concerning interpretation of data in an ATD is in order. First, the design does not control for the effects of extraneous variables in the experimental phase or the application phase. Although behavior increased during treatment, it is not possible to state unequivocally that the treatments were responsible for the increase. Even with alternation and counterbalancing the design is essentially an A-B design precluding strong statements about the variables responsible for behavioral changes. Many other variables could have been introduced simultaneously with the treatment and these variables may have influenced the behavior as much or more than the treatments. Similar limitations apply to the final phase with the added variable of sequence effects. Possibly, the behavior continues to improve principally because of the prior training rather than the current training. No controls for extraneous variables are present in either the experimental or application phase.

The lack of control is often overlooked in reporting study results, but it is a serious problem that must be taken into account in viewing results. Recognition of the problem prompted Kazdin and Hartmann (1978) to encourage applied researchers not to make absolute statements of treatment effectiveness, but only relative ones. It is safer to discuss differences between treatments when two are offered than to discuss effectiveness of treatment when treatment effects have not been isolated. Their advice is to refrain from using an alternating-treatments design to compare treatment versus no-treatment, and to restrict its use to comparing two or more treatments.

Naturally, all ATD studies do not conform strictly to the design in Figure 30. For instance, phase three is not essential. An investigator may choose to terminate the study after completing phase 2, the experimental phase. Others choose to use the third phase as an A phase as in an A-B-A design. The purpose of withdrawing all treatment in the final phase would be be to demonstrate control, that is, the treatments were responsible for the behavioral changes, not extraneous variables. It would be impossible to draw conclusions about which treatment effected the changes if both are withdrawn in the third phase. The most that could be said would be that when the two treatments were administered changes were obtained, but whether one treatment had a greater influence than the other cannot be examined. Indeed, the changes might have occurred only because both treatments were presented whereas either one alone would have been ineffective. Thus, planning a reversal for control is not designed for the purpose of issuing specific statements about specific treatments. Rather, it is designed to demonstrate that the treatments were successful.

Before discussing the strengths and weaknesses, the advantages and disadvantages of the alternating-treatments design, two examples of alternating-treatments studies are presented. One presents rather stable data that can be evaluated visually, whereas the other presents variable data necessitating statistical evaluation.

Murphy et al., (1979) entitled their study of cerebral palsy children "Multielement Designs: An Alternative to Reversal and Multiple Baseline Evaluation Strategies." Six nonambulatory, multihandicapped children in public school participated in the study. Two children had a diagnosis of spastic cerebral palsy and two hypotonic cerebral palsy. The purpose of the study was to attempt to increase upright head positioning by the children. The investigators used a photo-electric relay system to monitor head positioning. The two conditions compared were no-treatment and taped music contingent on upright head positioning.

Each session consisted of two 10–minute segments, a response-contingent reinforcement condition during which music was available, and the no-treatment, a baseline condition in which music was not available. When a lamp was lighted it signified that the contingent music condition was in effect and an unlighted lamp was associated with the no-treatment condition. The two conditions were alternated within each session. The order of presentation was counterbalanced so that each condition followed and was followed by the other condition equally often. The dependent variable consisted of the number of seconds per minute that each subject maintained an upright head position. Graphs for four children are presented in Figure 31. Results of the two conditions are clearest for Kathy and Ben. The contingent music treatment consistently resulted in a greater percentage of time with the head held up. There was no overlap between the two conditions. Clearly, the treatment was most effective for Ben, and although Kathy held her head up more and longer during the contingent music condition, the percent of time was still below 50% in all but one session. The music condition was also more effective in Bonnie's case with no overlap between treatments. Here again, however, the difference between conditions is not great, particularly in one of the later sessions, although the discrepancy is obvious in the last two sessions. The effectiveness of the contingent music treatment is least obvious in the results for Joan. Considerable variability occurred from session to session, the difference between the two conditions is small in some sessions and overlap

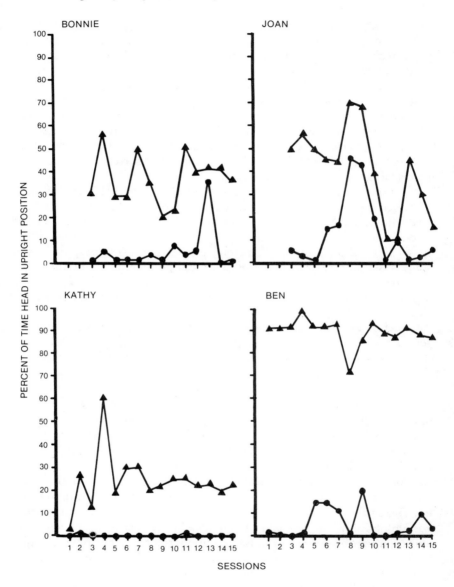

Figure 31. Percentage of time that subjects who initially exhibited little head control maintained their heads in a vertical position in no contingencies and contingent music conditions. *Circles* represent data from the portion of each session during which no contingencies were applied. *Triangles* represent data from the portion of each session during which contingent music was available. Missing data points indicate the subject was absent. (From Murphy et al., 1979, p. 25. Copyright by American Association on Mental Deficiency. Reproduced by permission).

occurred in session 12. It appeared that the effectiveness of treatment over no-treatment was not uniform across subjects, but the bulk of the evidence suggests that treatment is better than no-treatment.

The design of the study presented a problem, recognized and discussed by the authors, in that it was not possible to determine if the music functioned as a consequent event or simply as a stimulus that was present in one condition and not the other. In reality, as stated before, the ATD is essentially an A-B study so the influence of extraneous variables during the experimental phase was not controlled. Aside from that, the alternating-treatments design is well illustrated in the graphs of the children's behavior. Notice that there is no formal preexperimental baseline because one condition was a baseline. Additionally, the two conditions alternated within sessions rather than widely spaced time periods, making the separate baseline period even less essential. Neither was a final phase in which only contingent music was presented during the entire session included in the design. As mentioned, not all studies include a third phase.

The next was a more complex study with a number of variables that had to be accounted for. The study was conducted by Brady and Smouse (1978) and the design was labeled a *simultaneous-treatment design* by the investigators. A single subject was involved and the authors indicated that interaction and sequence effects were controlled by a Latin square design. Three treatments were compared for teaching an autistic child to follow a three-word instruction or request consisting of a noun, adjective, and verb, for example, "tap blue ring." The three treatments consisted of 1): vocalization (verbal instruction), 2) signing of the three-word commands, and 3) total communication for presenting the three-word instructions.

The behavior trained by the three treatments consisted of a nine-word language composed of three nouns, three verbs, and three adjectives. The words could be combined in a number of permutations to form different and novel commands. For example, "tap red block," "give red block," "Give blue block," and so on.

The three treatments were administered by three experimenters at three different time periods. The design was presented by the investigators in a table. The table for the counterbalanced arrangement is reproduced in Table 7. The design consisted of the three customary phases, baseline, three treatments, and implementation of the most effective treatment. In baseline, only verbal commands were used, as this constituted the dependent variable in the study. That is, regardless of how the child was trained, his responses to verbal requests were tested in novel sentence forms during and after training.

The variables needing counterbalancing were: 1) the three treatments, 2) the three experimenters, and 3) the three time periods in which the treatments were administered. Counterbalancing of treatments across time periods is clearly indicated. What is less clear in the table is whether the ex-

Table 7. Schematic representation of experimental design

Experimenter	Baseline phase	Simultaneous treatment phase			Final phase
		Block 1 (Sessions 1–7)	Block 2 (Sessions 8–14)	Block 3 (Sessions 15–21)	
1	Verbalization	Verbalization	Signing	Simultaneous communication	Simultaneous communication
2	Verbalization	Signing	Simultaneous communication	Verbalization	Simultaneous communication
3	Verbalization	Simultaneous communication	Verbalization	Signing	Simultaneous communication

From Brady and Smouse, 1978, p. 276. Copyright by Plenum Publishing Corp. Reproduced by permission.

perimenters were also alternated in time periods. That is, according to the table it appears that experimenter 1 always administered treatment first, followed by experimenter 2, and then experimenter 3. If this was true, then the study was partially, not totally counterbalanced. A total counterbalancing would entail the design shown in Table 8. The experimenters may have accounted for all possible permutations and it simply is not characterized in the table. Recall Kazdin and Hartmann's (1978) admonishment that the more treatments and the more variables changed in the stimulus condition, the more complex the design becomes. The 9 days shown in the table would be insufficient for a study because each order would be presented only once. Thus additional days would be needed to allow the subject to differentiate the treatments from the experimenters and time periods and to allow training to take place.

Results of the study by Brady and Smouse (1978) are presented in Figure 32. The three phases of the study are separated by vertical lines. The first observation in examining the data from the last two phases is the variability in the child's responses and the overlap in the data during the simultaneous-treatment phase. A visual examination of the data would lead one to conclude that no one treatment stands out as most effective. Statistics were used to evaluate treatment effectiveness. White's (1972) method of fitting a median trend line and a simple binomial test was used after it had been determined the special Latin square analysis of variance (Benjamin, 1965) was inappropriate. Comparison did not involve a comparison of the three treatments among themselves, but rather each respective treatment result was compared to the baseline measure. The total-communication procedure was revealed as more effective than either the vocal or the signing procedure when measured against baseline. Therefore, the total-communication procedure was administered by all experimenters across all time periods in phase three. Here, too, the data demonstrate considerable variability, a range from 21 correct to 5 correct responses.

The study has several important components of the alternating-treatments or simultaneous-treatment design, mainly counterbalancing, alternation, and the three phases considered appropriate to the design. Other features were also well planned. It is unusual, however, to compare each

Table 8. A schematic for counterbalancing three treatments, three experimenters and three time periods

Time period	Days								
	1	2	3	4	5	6	7	8	9
a	E_1-T_1	E_1-T_2	E_1-T_3	E_2-T_1	E_2-T_2	E_2-T_3	E_3-T_1	E_3-T_2	E_3-T_3
b	E_2-T_2	E_2-T_3	E_2-T_1	E_3-T_2	E_3-T_3	E_3-T_1	E_1-T_2	E_1-T_3	E_1-T_1
c	E_3-T_3	E_3-T_1	E_3-T_2	E_1-T_3	E_1-T_1	E_1-T_2	E_2-T_3	E_2-T_1	E_2-T_2

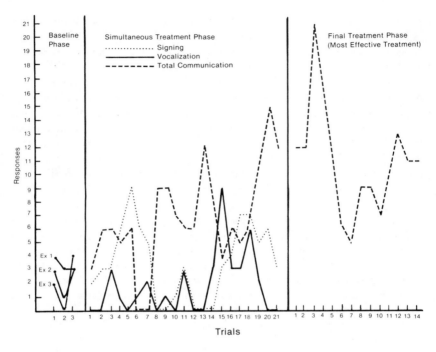

Figure 32. Frequency of correct responses to experimental language across all phases. (From Brady and Smouse, 1978, p. 277. Copyright by Plenum Publishing Corp. Reproduced by permission).

treatment with baseline instead of comparing treatments with each other, because that is the intent of the design. Need for statistical analysis of the data to tease out differences between treatments and baseline is obvious because visual examination would lead to the conclusion that 1) the treatments were not wholly effective and that 2) consistency of treatment effects was not obtained irrespective of the treatment. Whether one wishes to accept the authors' conclusions regarding the effectiveness of total communication on the basis of the statistical test and the data that were compared, after viewing the raw data in the graph, is a decision each investigator makes. Regardless, the conclusions must still be considered somewhat tentative simply because the ATD does not control for extraneous variables during the second and third phases.

As mentioned, variations of the basic design have been reported in the applied research literature. Counterbalancing in some is minimal, the number of phases differ, and dependence on statistical treatments of the data varies. As yet, the design is not used widely, particularly for communicative disorders research, so the sample is small. Its usefulness in investigation of differences in treatments has not been clearly demonstrated, but the promise is there. To help investigators make decisions regarding the use of alternating-treatments designs a section on advantages and disadvantages associated with the design (and related designs) follows.

Additional Considerations

An important question in communicative disorders treatment concerns the effectiveness of a treatment. With a multitude of treatment variables and treatment packages available, the clinician is hard pressed at times to decide which treatment is most appropriate for a given client. Little experimental effort has been directed to comparing two or more treatments claimed to be effective in treating a particular disorder or communicative behavior. Yet, for example, as the Code of Ethics of the American Speech-Language-Hearing Association (1980) directs, intervention variables and programs must be evaluated in a controlled fashion. The alternating-treatments design offers a vehicle for examining differences in clinical procedures, an evaluation the traditional A-B-A-B or multiple-baseline designs cannot readily accomplish. Even the more complex interaction designs cannot be used to compare two treatments administered concurrently. In fact, in some aspects the ATD offers a sophisticated and elegant way to compare treatments because subject variables, which usually present serious confounding problems, are not present. The subject serves as his own control receiving both treatments. If a subject characteristic affects one treatment, it will also influence the other, thereby eliminating subject variables as a possible confound. Other variables, such as passage of time, are also held constant because the treatments are administered concurrently. Appropriately designed, therefore, the ATD provides a framework for comparing treatments, a much-neglected, but much-needed endeavor in communicative disorders. As long as the limitations of the design for exploring treatment effectiveness are recognized, the ATD can provide useful information concerning relative strengths of two or more treatments.

Like the multiple-baseline design, the ATD can be employed when the behavior treated is irreversible or a reversal is undesirable. Staff members in schools or institutions are more comfortable with rapid alternation of baseline and treatment or treatments than of the long reversal phase in an A-B-A-B study (Ulman and Sulzer-Azaroff, 1975; Barlow and Hayes, 1979; Hersen and Barlow, 1976). After all, a return to baseline in an ATD lasts only one session at a time because the subject is receiving treatment every other session. For all concerned, the situation is less aversive than a reversal.

Time saved is another advantage often mentioned. Because the conditions are alternated rapidly the study is completed in less time. In an A-B-A-B design, the phases, each several sessions in length, are presented in sequence, customarily a time-consuming project. Inasmuch as the second baseline in a multiple-baseline design must await termination or at least a reasonable period of training on the first baseline, it too is time consuming. The problem is compounded in interaction designs that require a greater number of phases in sequence. The ATD takes less time because treatments are not presented one after the other; they are presented concurrently in alternation. True, investigators propose a phase for administering the most effective treatment, but it is not essential for answering questions about the treatments in the experimental phase. A third phase adds length to a study, but with or without it the ATD can be used with an eye to time conservation. Unlike the A-B-A-B or multiple-baseline study, the entire study need not be conducted in order to obtain useful data (Ulman and Sulzer-Azaroff, 1975; Barlow and Hayes, 1979). Comparison data begin to accumulate from the first treatment day. Even if the study is aborted after several sessions, the investigator has comparison data on the conditions. With an A-B-A-B or multiple-baseline study, the design requires completion of all phases before data are analyzed for treatment effects.

It is often noted that unstable baselines need not concern the investigator. This would be true only in the treatment/no-treatment study in which baseline is measured in alternation with treatment. In this study, instability would be a problem only if the treatment data overlapped with the baseline data. Variability in the treatment data, or overlap in the baseline and treatment data would hinder interpretation of results. When two treatments are compared, a stable baseline is as essential as in an A-B-A-B or multiple-baseline study.

A possible shortcoming for communicative disorders research is that the alternating-treatments design may have greater applicability for evaluating treatments of on-off behaviors, for example, disruptive behaviors, than of behaviors learned gradually in treatment. For the most part, behaviors involved in communicative disorders fall into the latter group. Disfluency would be amenable to evaluation of two concurrent treatments, articulation less so. Correcting error sounds requires a procedure in which approximations are shaped into correct productions. If two treatments were compared, the sound may have been approximated during the first treatment, improved when treatment 2 was initiated and correct production achieved during the next session when treatment one was readministered. Evaluating the individual contributions of the two treatments would not be possible. Thus, behaviors learned in stages would more likely be vulnerable to confounding than behaviors defined as simply present or absent in the subject's repertoire (sitting or not sitting).

Another weakness of the alternating-treatments design is the possibility of multiple-treatment interference. Two kinds of interference may occur: sequential effects and carry-over effects (Barlow and Hayes, 1979; Ulman and Sulzer-Azaroff, 1975; Kratochwill and Levin, 1980; Kazdin and Hartmann, 1978; Hersen and Barlow, 1976). Of the two, researchers are better acquainted with sequential effects.

Investigators are accustomed to controlling for order effects when administration of one independent variable follows another in either within-subject or group experimental designs. If proper measures are not taken, effects of a treatment on the effectiveness of subsequent treatments cannot be ruled out. That is to say, when two or more treatments are involved, behavioral changes cannot be attributed to any one treatment unless each treatment is preceded and followed by the other treatment(s). Otherwise, changes could be a function of the prior treatment(s). Order, or sequencing effects, are controlled by counterbalancing treatments, a topic discussed at length in earlier sections of this book. Owing to the purpose of the design, counterbalancing is an integral component of alternating-treatments studies. In addition to administration of treatments, other variables are counterbalanced if they threaten to interfere with isolation of the effect of a treatment. Sequence effects are controlled through counterbalancing.

Carry-over effects are less amenable to control in ATD studies. Investigators have identified two kinds of carry-over effects: contrast and induction. Incidentally, differences between sequencing and carry-over effects are not easily defined. The difference appears to be in the extent of the effect. In sequence effects, each treatment in a sequence will cumulatively affect subsequent treatments. Thus, treatment 1 has an effect on treatment 2, and treatments 1 and 2 effect treatment 3, and so forth. Carry-over effects, on the other hand, are anlayzed in terms of adjacent phases or treatments only, that is, the immediately preceding or following treatment.

Contrast effects are present when a behavior in treatment changes in a direction opposite to what is expected due to the contrast with an adjacent treatment (Barlow and Hayes, 1979). The example commonly offered is of two punishment conditions. If a 1–minute time-out treatment follows a 15–minute time-out treatment, the 1–minute time-out, instead of serving as a mild punisher, could function as a reinforcer (Azrin and Holz, 1966). If so, the 1–minute time-out treatment would have an opposite effect on the behavior from the effect it would have if it were not preceded by the 15–minute time-out treatment. In a similar vein, if fluency were consequated by a hug, a smile, and verbal praise in one treatment and in the following condition fluency resulted only in a brief smile, the brief smile might serve as a mild punisher in contrast to the previous lavish treatment, whereas normally it would be expected to function as a reinforcer.

Conversely, in induction a treatment is enhanced when preceded by another treatment. Accordingly, behavior in treatment 2 resembles the behavior obtained in treatment 1 more than would be anticipated if treatment 2 had been administered without treatment 1. Barlow and Hayes (1979) note that if the 1–minute time-out period resulted in a greater decrease in behavior when following the 15–minute time-out period than when preceding it, induction would have occurred. By the same token, if the auxiliary verb form is acquired in fewer trials following copula training than when it is the only training administered, or when it precedes copula training, the investigator would suspect induction from one treatment to another.

Investigators are encouraged to be alert to the two kinds of carry-over effects in applied research. This is not to say that it is necessary to assume their presence in all ATD studies. Nonetheless, when they appear likely, the experimenter takes them into account, qualifying results and conclusions accordingly. Fortunately, the effects, when present, have not been found to be great (Ulman and Sulzer-Azaroff, 1975; Barlow and Hayes, 1979). It should be pointed out that controls have been developed for sequence effects in single-subject and group studies, but less attention has been paid to carry-over effects. Several solutions for overcoming carry-over effects have been proposed.

The most obvious solution is counterbalancing. Not only does counterbalancing help eliminate sequencing effects, it can also help rule out contrast and/or induction. If each treatment precedes and follows the other treatments without appearance of a pattern in behavioral changes as a function of any two adjacent treatments, the possibility of carry-over effects may be dismissed.

Other procedures can be incorporated into the study design to prevent carry-over effects. First, the two treatments can be separated from each other by a reasonable time period. For example, instead of presenting one treatment in the first half and another in the last half of a session, present only one treatment per session, for example, one in the morning, and one in the afternoon. Keeping in mind that the two treatments should not be widely spaced from each other, after all, fast alternation is one of the strengths of the alternating-treatments design, plan an interval that is reasonable but will not decrease the efficiency of the design.

Another suggestion concerns the rapidity with which treatments or conditions are alternated. The speedier the alternation, the more probable are carry-over effects. Again, the investigator must consider all factors in scheduling alternations. If they are too slow, advantages inherent in fast alternation are weakened, whereas if too fast, the subject may not discriminate between treatments. A careful investigator gives judicious thought to procedures enhancing control of multiple-treatment interference.

Another solution to carry-over effects is obtaining direct data on contrast and induction through evaluation of each treatment in isolation and within the alternating-treatments design (Barlow and Hayes, 1979; Sidman, 1960). Two procedures are offered: independent verification and functional manipulation.

In independent verification, the experimenter explores each treatment individually in an A-B design. Comparison involves observing each treatment presented alone and presented alternatively with other treatments. If two treatments were involved, evaluation would require a minimum of three verifications. Treatment A would be administered alone in an A-B design. It would also be administered as one of the treatments in the ATD study. Treatment B would be handled in a similar manner. If no differences were found between a treatment presented individually and in alternation, carry-over effects need not be a strong concern. Needless to say, results would require qualification because the verification occurred in an A-B format, disallowing cause and effect statements.

In functional manipulation, the experimenter changes the strength of one of the treatments. Perhaps the selected treatment is carried out for a longer period, or at a greater intensity and frequency. In this procedure, quantitative differences for short periods are programmed. Thus, one treatment might consist of 2 seconds of noise for a low intensity voice and the second of a 2–second blast of air for the same behavior. For several sessions the intensity of the noise is increased and then returned to the original intensity. If the change is followed by a change in behavior during the treatment not manipulated, the intensity change in the first treatment might have been responsible. The shift in behavior in the unmanipulated treatment could be evidence of carry-over effects.

Both of the above procedures are possible, but either one would add length to the study. Recall that one of the advantages of the ATD is that it is less time consuming. Adding two A-B phases (more with replication) lessens the attractiveness of the alternating-treatments design. Neither is it clear what information would be obtained in isolating a treatment in an A-B portion. An A-B design, as frequently pointed out, is a descriptive, not an experimental design. Effectiveness of a treatment requires a controlled evaluation, as in an A-B-A study. As for the functional manipulation procedure, changing duration, frequency, or intensity of one treatment may also change the study, confounding it by not providing equal opportunity to all treatments. An important factor in the ATD is that the treatments be presented equally often, and we assume that equality also applies to length of time and intensity of treatment. The solutions for exploring carry-over effects promise to complicate ATD studies.

In addition to sequential and carry-over effects, Barlow and Hayes (1979) add alternation effects as a concern in designing alternating-treatments studies. Possibly, rapidly alternating two treatments could be more effective than administering either intervention alone. The important factor is rapid alternation, irrespective of treatments. Barlow and Hayes (1979) speculate that this may represent an intensification of treatment effects owing to a sharpening of stimulus control. To study this possibility an investigator could "alternate" periods of fast alternations with periods of slower alternations to determine if differences are found.

An investigator who is aware of the possible confounds present in treatment-comparison studies is able to recognize the effects. Presently, the extent of carry-over effects in ATD studies is conjectural. The proposed solutions have rarely been implemented to explore contrast, induction, and alternation effects. Nevertheless, evidence for contrast effects was obtained in a study by Koegel, Egel, and Williams (1980) to be described briefly. Three autistic children participated. The target behavior for child 1 was compliance with instructions (e.g., "bring me the spoon"). For the other two children, attending to the object specified by the experimenter was the target behavior. The design was described as a multiple-baseline design across subjects, but child 1's treatment sessions were alternated with no-treatment sessions. Procedures for child 2 included 30 trials on the average each day, beginning either with a treatment or no-treatment period on a random schedule. Only child 3 was not administered treatment and no-treatment on an alternating schedule. For all children, intervention consisted of praise for correct responses accompanied by food and a verbal "no" for incorrect responses. No consequent events were administered for responses in the no-treatment periods.

Before treatment, baseline measures of varying lengths were taken for each child. The target behaviors in both the treatment setting and no-treatment setting were counted. During baseline, the target behaviors occurred at a moderate rate. When treatment was initiated, the target behaviors increased above baseline levels in the treatment setting as expected. Unexpectedly, they decreased below baseline levels in the no-treatment settings. The investigators suggested that the results demonstrated contrast effects because the behavior changed in the no-treatment (extended baseline) condition when treatment was initiated. They point out that the treatment consisted of highly discriminable reinforcement contingencies that functioned to make the contrast between treatment and no-treatment settings obvious, thereby depressing the behavior in all but the treatment condition.

The results lend support to the presence of contrast effects in comparing treatments. Of course, the study was not designed as an alternating-treatments design and this should be weighed in considering the results. For example, treatment was always administered in one setting and no-treatment (extra therapy) in another setting. One adult administered the treatment while another tested the target behavior. Nevertheless, the study indicates that carry-over effects might occur when two treatments are compared. To counter the possibility, it would be well to plan on obtaining objective data demonstrating that carry-over effects are not present.

Although not necessarily a problem in the ATD, the manner in which the data are analyzed and presented constitutes an issue. In all likelihood, communicative disorders research will lend itself infrequently to clearcut data on the superiority of one treatment over another. More often, comparison may result in data reflecting overlap and/or moderate to wide variation in the treatments evaluated, making interpretation of results difficult. The variability may force investigators to choose between using inferential statistics and relying on visual graphing in analyzing and interpreting data. Kratochwill and Levin (1980) note that most alternating-treatments and simultaneous-treatment design studies employ inferential statistical tests to complement visual inspection of results. They caution, however, against using parametric analysis of variance procedures, suggesting that within-subject designs require different statistical treatment from that used for large sample studies. Application of statistics not developed specifically for $N = 1$ repeated measures studies violates the assumptions underlying them and leads to invalid conclusions. If statistical procedures are employed, selecting appropriate procedures is important to avoid erroneous conclusions regarding treatment effectiveness.

The option is the investigator's—reliance on visual inspection or statistical treatment. The option may be converted to a decision between adopting clinical or statistical criteria to evaluate treatment effects. Though the ATD appears to be amenable to, or perhaps more needful of, statistical treatment, the issue is no different from using statistics for evaluating data in any single-subject intervention designs. Certainly a compromise is available: when effects are large, visual inspection is chosen; when variability obscures results, statistics are used (Kratochwill and Levin, 1980). We would avoid statistical procedures and compromise, opting for visual inspection for the same reasons we chose it for other within-subject designs. Briefly stated, if the effects are so small that they need to be teased out by statistical procedures, are they clincally relevant?

Naturally, investigators will differ in their choices of data analysis. Hopefully, those selecting statistical treatment will also present the raw data so that each viewer can reach his or her own decision regarding differences between treatments. Presenting both forms of data would allow independent decisions about the usefulness of the treatments to specific clients.

Before leaving the topic of alternating-treatments design, a word or two about designs used either interchangeably with, or resembling, the ATD will be included. Basically, there is agreement on the function of the designs, but agreement on the exact components in each is lacking. No attempt will be made to reconcile the differences; rather, each design is described in general terms. Most of the designs have not been used in communicative disorders research. Hopefully, as they become more common in other behavioral research, communicative disorders researchers will start adapting them to investigations of speech, language, and hearing.

Multiple-Schedule Design

According to Barlow and Hayes (1979) the term *multiple schedule* implies association of a distinct schedule with each of several stimuli. The design had its origin in basic research (Sidman, 1960). More than one intervention can be evaluated with the design. Kazdin and Hartmann (1978) explain that in the design each intervention is associated with a particular stimulus. The purpose is to demonstrate that behavior comes under the control of the specific stimulus with which each intervention is associated. Alternation is not necessary (Kazdin and Hartmann, 1978), but is sometimes included. Hersen and Barlow (1976), in comparing the multiple-baseline with the multiple-schedule design, explain that, whereas in the multiple-baseline design independent behaviors are treated individually in sequence, in the multiple-schedule design the same behavior is treated differentially under varying stimulus conditions. Leitenberg (1973) points out that the multiple-schedule design involves discrimination learning, in that if the same behavior is treated differently in the presence of different physical or social stimuli, it will show different characteristics when the stimuli are present. The discriminative stimuli might consist of different time periods, settings, or therapists. Examples of multiple-schedule designs in applied behavior analysis research cited by Hersen and Barlow (1976) include studies by O'Brien, Azrin and Henson (1969), Agras et al. (1969), and Wahler (1969). The studies contain some of the components included in descriptions of ATD studies, but also differ in other respects.

Multielement-Baseline Design

Ulman and Sulzer-Azaroff (1975) describe a design identical to the alternating-treatments design proposed by Barlow and Hayes (1979) with a different label. The name they chose to use is the *Multielement-Baseline Design*. Barlow and Hayes' preference for *alternating-treatments design* is explained by reference to Sidman's (1960) original application of the term *multielement baseline* to studies designed to investigate the effect of a single condition on more than one behavior. The authors remark that, conversely, the ATD is designed to investigate the effect of more than one condition on a single behavior. Ulman and Sulzer-Azaroff (1975), recognizing the similarity in the two designs, comment that *alternating-conditions design* could replace their label *multielement-baseline design*. The only difference mentioned is that *multielement baseline* emphasizes behavioral effects, whereas *alternating conditions* emphasizes experimental conditions. Barlow and Hayes (1979) agree with this position preferring to call attention to the experimental conditions in using the term *alternating-treatments design*. As nearly as can be determined, therefore, the two labels refer to the same design as evidenced in the studies reported in the literature under the name *multielement-baseline design*. Following Barlow and Hayes (1979) suggestion, we chose to call the design *alternating-treatments design*.

Randomization Design

The randomization design developed by Edgington (1967, 1972) is also capable of comparing treatments in a controlled manner. The design was not developed from operant psychology in that treatments are deliberately randomized across time periods. Each treatment is repeated often enough to allow statistical comparison of treatments (e.g., A-B-B-A-B-A-A). Because the design was developed to enable statistical evaluation it will not be discussed further as a within-subject design in the context of the definition used herein.

The Simultaneous-Treatment Design

The name *simultaneous-treatment design* is probably used most often as a synonym for studies qualifying as *alternating-treatments design*. Hersen and Barlow (1976) also refer to it as a *concurrent-schedule design*. They explain that "...in the concurrent schedule strategy the subject is *simultaneously* exposed to different stimulus conditions" (p. 258). Although other investigators do not make the distinction, Barlow and Hayes (1979) contend that the difference between the alternating-treatments design and simultaneous-treatment design is that in the latter the treatments are actually available at the same time. Therefore, the procedure becomes a preference procedure with the subject choosing the preferred treatment. When this occurs, the treatments are naturally administered an unequal number of times because the subject approaches the procedure preferred. Unequal exposure to treatments violates an important component of the alternating-treatments design, therefore, the two designs are different and function differently. Kazdin and Hartmann (1978), however, do not concur with the description. They state that:

> The simultaneous-treatment design also examines different interventions that are implemented in an "alternating" fashion. However, the interventions are balanced across stimulus conditions (e.g., time periods, situations, agents and treatments) so that the effects of different interventions are unconfounded by the different stimulus conditions. (p. 914).

The description is identical to a description of an ATD study. Nevertheless, as pointed out by Barlow and Hayes (1979) the original simultaneous-treatment design study by Browning (1967) did present the treatments simultaneously. Examination of the procedural descriptions provided by Browning (1967) and again by Browning and Stover (1971) did not help to clarify this point. The procedures were not described specifically enough to determine whether treatments were alternated or presented simultaneously. Regardless, most investigators have used an alternating design when the study has been labeled a simultaneous-treatment design. Therefore, the two designs seem to be identical, as were the multielement-baseline design and the alternating-treatments design.

We will turn now to another category of designs that can be used to evaluate the effects of more than one independent variable in a treatment. According to Hersen and Barlow (1976), the designs enable investigation of interaction effects in treatments composed of more than one component.

INTERACTION DESIGNS

Interaction designs do not compare treatments in the same sense as alternating-treatments designs do because they take the A-B-A form in which phases follow each other in sequence. In fact, the purpose of an interaction design is to evaluate additive, subtractive, that is, interactive effects of individual components of a treatment rather than comparison of two treatments. This means that the treatment consists of more than one variable, for example, "good" for correct responses and "no" for incorrect responses. Any statements regarding the effectiveness of "good" alone, or "no" alone require that each be evaluated separately and in the context of the other. If "good" were treatment B, and "no" treatment C, the entire package would be labeled BC. Without evaluation of the individual contribution of B and of C the design would follow the classic A-B-A design, except that the treatment portion would specify the existence of two variables. Thus, the design would be represented as an A-BC-A-BC design. If the investigator wished to study the contributions of B and C and the interactive effects of both, however, each variable would be evaluated alone and in conjunction with the other. The design might take the form of A-B-BC-B-BC if the separate contribution of B is of interest. In this design the effect of B alone is tested first. Then the effect of B and C administered together is examined; and returning to B alone completes a controlled evaluation. The final BC is not essential but follows the more acceptable A-B-A-B design format.

Several important principles need to be kept in mind in evaluating treatment components in interaction designs. The one-variable rule applies. Only one variable is manipulated at a time as in any A-B-A study. Each variable to be evaluated must be adjacent to the rest. Thus, an A-BC-A-B design would not be appropriate for evaluating the B component alone and in interaction with C. Why? First, the components evaluated are not adjacent to each other, they are separated by an A phase. Comparison of the behavior in B with the behavior in BC is interfered with because of the intervening A phase. Second, the additive or subtractive effects of B can be evaluated only in the context of the controlled A-B-A format. The B-BC-B design supplies the necessary controls for ruling out confounding variables, whereas the BC-A-B design does not. In summary, unless the components are in adjacent phases and in the basic A-B-A design, an investigator cannot discuss the effects of either component alone or in contrast to the total treatment package. In a B-BC-B design, the B phases serve as baseline for BC, allowing the analysis of additive and controlling effects.

An error frequently made by investigators is evaluation of components in sequence with baseline intervening between treatments. The design would be A-B-A-C. Needless to say, investigators using these designs neglect to consider confounding due to order or sequence effects. Whatever occurs in C could be confounded by the treatment in B and effects of C cannot be evaluated. Even if counterbalancing is used by administering an A-C-A-B sequence to another subject, statements concerning the effectiveness of the combination of the two variables are not possible with an A-B-A-C / A-C-A-B design because the two have never been combined to determine if the combination is different from the two in sequence. That is, the effects of B and C over A can be evaluated but the relative or combined effects of B and C cannot.

To reiterate, in interaction designs the interactive effects of two or more variables can be examined. This is accomplished by examining the effects of both variables alone and in combination. The analysis goes beyond the analysis of the separate effects of more than one variable over baseline, as in an A-B-A-C design (Hersen and Barlow, 1976).

Another design often interpreted as revealing interactive and relative effects is the A-B-A-B-BC design. It is totally inadequate for the purpose. The final two phases (B-BC) form an uncontrolled A-B design and is descriptive, not experimental in nature.

The realization that it is not possible to discuss relative effectiveness of two or more components from an A-B-A-C study has not come to many investigators. The majority of studies evaluating the relative effects of separate treatment components use the inappropriate A-B-A-C design, in which comparison with baseline only is possible.

It is possible to design an interaction study for evaluating more than two variables, but the design would become quite complex and cumbersome. To explore the additive and interactive effects of three components, the following design would be required: A-B-BCD-B-BCD; C-BCD-C-BCD; D-BCD-D-BCD. Obviously, the design becomes so complex that the study seems prohibitive. Yet, if controlled evaluations of treatment components is the goal, that is what would be required for a treatment package of three components.

On the other hand, if an investigator is not concerned about the contributions of separate components, an interaction design is not required. Instead, the design would be the simple A-BCD-A-BCD design in which the entire treatment package is evaluated in total. As long as the investigator does not attribute specific effects to specific components, the design is adequate. The most to be said is that the program is effective as it is.

At times the A and B phases are collapsed. This occurs when the B variable produces no change in the behavior after baseline. When the data from baseline and B phases are comparable, the two phases are collapsed into an extended A phase. The treatment in B was shown to be ineffective alone.

A variation of the interaction design includes starting with a complete treatment package subtracting one of the components and then replacing it. The design would be A-BC-B-BC-B. It is really no different from the other regarding phases in sequence, except that it begins with the entire treatment program.

In Table 9, the designs in use, complete and incomplete, are listed. Properly designed interactive studies are complex designs and require several subjects to complete.

Good examples of interaction design studies are not available in the communicative disorders literature and are also scarce in any within-subject intervention research. We have selected one example from a classroom study because it conforms nicely to the requirements of the interaction design. The other was selected from communicative disorders research because it demonstrates the commonly used design for exploring relative effectiveness of treatments. It is not an interaction design, but has often been so interpreted in the research literature.

Table 9. Complete and incomplete interaction designs to study relative effectiveness of single components and combinations of components

Design	Changes	Status
A-B-BC-B-BC	add B or C	Complete
A-BC-B-BC-B	subtract B or C	Complete
A-B-A-C		Incomplete
A-B-A-BC		Incomplete
A-BC-A-B		Incomplete
A-BC-A-BC		Not interactive

The A-B-BC-B-BC study was conducted by Frank Gresham (1979) and was entitled "Comparison of response cost and timeout in a special education setting." The study concerned methods that could be used to decrease rate of noncompliance in a group of educable mentally retarded children in a public school. The two treatments, consisting of time-out and response cost, were evaluated in relation to effectiveness of each variable independently and in interaction.

Noncompliance was defined as a child not complying with a teacher's command within 5 seconds after it had been presented. The commands consisted of telling each child to go to a particular area for a specific activity. The experimental design consisted of a baseline, response cost$_1$, response cost plus time-out$_1$, response cost$_2$, and response cost plus time-out$_2$. The study was designed to allow the experimenter to draw conclusions regarding the relative effectiveness of response cost and time-out, as well as to assess the interaction of both procedures in decreasing rates of noncompliance.

After a 7-day baseline in which no contingencies were in effect, Phase B, response cost, was put into effect for 5 days. Noncompliance with teacher commands resulted in a loss of tokens that the children normally earned for classroom activities. In Phase BC, response cost plus time-out, the child not only lost a token for noncompliance (response cost) but was required to sit in a chair outside the group (time-out) for 1 minute. The phase lasted 6 days. Phase B$_2$, response cost, was identical to Phase B$_1$ and lasted 5 days. Phase BC$_2$, response cost plus time-out, continued for 5 days. A 5–day follow-up phase, conducted 3 months after completion, was included in the study. The results are presented in Figure 33.

Averaged data across subjects is presented in the figure. Clearly, the changes in noncompliance across phases are not dramatic. However, shifts in the average number of responses occurred; 48% in baseline, 11% in response cost$_1$, 13% in the combined response cost plus time-out, and 5% in the second response cost phase. In the final combined treatment phase, noncompliance rose to 12%. Shifts among the phases were evaluated by t-tests. Comparisons were made between baseline and response cost phases, and baseline and the two response cost plus time-out phases. All of these comparisons revealed significant differences. However, the comparison between response cost alone and response cost plus time-out showed no significant difference. On the basis of the comparisons, the investigator concluded that response cost alone was as effective as the combined treatment. Visual inspection of the data does not lead to obvious conclusions regarding the results. The strongest evidence is in the BC-B-BC sequence and, although the differences are small and the behavior variable, the data present the possibility that response cost was equally as effective as the combination in BC. Although the differences between B and BC are not readily observed, the

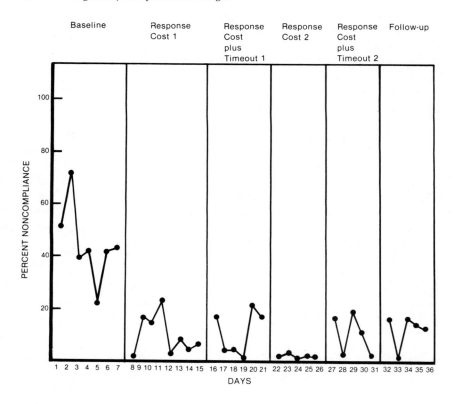

Figure 33. Daily average of noncompliance to teacher commands. (From Gresham, 1979, p. 204. Copyright by Buttonwood Forms, Inc. Reproduced by permission).

study illustrates the form of an interaction design for exploring more than one treatment.

A more common method for exploring relative effectiveness of more than one treatment in communicative disorders is presentation of several treatments in sequence, either in alternation with baseline phases, as in the Costello and Ferrer (1976) study, or with no baseline phases between treatment phases, as in the Engel and Groth (1976) study discussed in Chapter 4.

A sequential study in which baseline phases alternated with treatments was conducted by Costello and Hairston (1976). The study was not designed to examine interactive effects, and the authors make no such claim. The study is discussed here only because the design is so frequently used by investigators to evaluate interactive effects, an improper design for this purpose. Costello and Hairston (1976) did not use the design in that manner.

In Costello and Hairston's (1976) study, several consequent events were used to "punish" incorrect articulation responses and off-task behaviors during articulation training. The conditions in effect across phases consisted of the following: reponse cost for both incorrect articulation and off-task behaviors; response cost for incorrect articulation and buzzer for off-task behaviors; buzzer for incorrect productions and for each off-task behavior; buzzer for each incorrect articulation and response cost for each off-task behavior. The treatments were administered across phases with a no-punishment condition between each punishment condition. If response cost is designated as treatment B, the buzzer as treatment C, and the no-punishment condition as A, the design would be specified as an A-B-A-BC-A-C-A-BC-A design. Three treatment conditions were included; response cost alone, buzzer alone, and buzzer and response cost combined. The treatments were administered in various combinations for incorrect articulation responses and off-task behaviors. Thus, there was an intermingling of treatment effects across behaviors and phases. During the study, the sound receiving training changed across phases as did the treatment program. We will not dwell on these variables, however, because it is the design that is of interest in this chapter. Results for the articulation training are presented in Figure 34. Because the data for the off-task behaviors were similar they will not be presented.

The variability in behavior within phases does not allow clear-cut interpretation of the data, but the most important point for the purpose of this discussion is that a baseline phase is inserted between each treatment phase. Therefore, comparisons can be made between each individual treatment and no-treatment conditions, but not between treatments. The A phases interspersed between each treatment condition indicate that the study was not an interaction design that would require adjacent treatment phases and the B-BC-B (A-B-A) control. The authors wisely refrain from statements regarding comparison of treatments and refer only to the differences between no-punishment and punishment conditions. They also observe rightly that sequence effects were probably operating in the last four phases, in that incorrect articulation responses decreased and remained at a lower level of frequency regardless of the condition in effect. It is not possible, of course, to attribute the results entirely to the treatments, because the sounds being trained and the complexity of the training steps were also changing across phases. The investigators recognized the possible confusion in their discussion of results.

To develop an interaction design, the following sequence of phases would be necessary in order to evaluate both response cost and buzzer individually as they interact: A-B-BC-B-BC:A-C-BC-C-BC. It would probably also be easier to explore effects of the two procedures on the two behaviors in

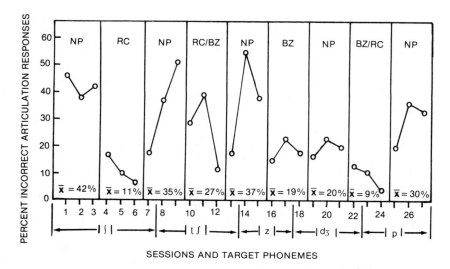

Figure 34. Percentage of incorrect articulation responses for each session within each experimental condition: NP, nonpunishment; RC, response cost applied to both incorrect articulation and off-task behaviors; RC/BZ, response cost applied to incorrect articulation and buzzer applied to off-task behaviors; BZ, buzzer applied to both groups of behavior; BZ/RC, buzzer for incorrect articulation and response cost for off-task behaviors. The average percent of incorrect responses for each condition is indicated as are phonemes being treated across sessions. (From Costello and Hairston, 1976, p. 182. Copyright by American Elsevier Publishing Company, Inc. Reproduced by permission).

individual studies, one for each behavior, rather than incorporating both in one study.

Additional Considerations

Intervention evaluation is an important aspect of applied behavior research. As the number of treatment variables and treatments increases, comparisons between treatments assume a higher priority. The alternating-treatments and interaction designs provide alternative strategies and tactics for examining treatment components. Both have weaknesses and strengths. The one to be used depends upon the question posed by the investigator. If treatments are to be compared, ATD is more appropriate than the interaction design. But if a treatment package is available and an investigator wishes to determine how well each component functions in the package, the interaction design suits better.

The interaction design has some of the problems of the classic A-B-A-B design in that all phases need to be completed and it is time consuming. The more components examined, the longer it takes to complete the study. The length adds to the basic time-locked problem in A-B-A-B studies because additional phases are required. There is some danger of sequence effects as one phase follows another. Counterbalancing and replication are required, meaning that the subject population would be increased. Although most investigators choose to examine treatment components without subtracting or adding the components singly from the package, the interaction design offers a more efficient means for eliminating irrelevant procedures and preserving strong ones. The result would be treatment programs consisting only of the most effective procedures. Without interaction designs, an investigator can address the issue of comparing treatments with baseline, but not the contribution of components within treatments. Additional designs allowing for an in-depth evaluation of treatment components are presented next.

As noted above, practical considerations may limit the use of designs that assess the relative effectiveness of intervention techniques and many investigators will continue to explore individual treatment strategies. Furthermore, in addition to comparing treatment techniques and evaluating the overall efficacy of multifaceted intervention packages, applied researchers may want to evaluate the appropriateness of individual steps within a treatment program or determine the success of various shaping procedures. Two within-subject experimental strategies that can be used to investigate these and related issues, the changing-criterion and multiple-probe designs are considered in the sections that follow.

CHANGING-CRITERION DESIGN

The changing-criterion design is a variation of the multiple-baseline design that can be used to evaluate the effects of treatment on a single, gradually acquired behavior and it is particularly appropriate for studying the effectiveness of shaping procedures (Hartmann and Hall, 1976; Hall and Fox, 1977). There are two primary experimental phases in a changing-criterion design; a baseline and a treatment phase. During the baseline phase, a single behavior is monitored over time until a stable response rate is achieved. Baseline performance is subsequently used to establish an initial criterion level and treatment is initiated until the target behavior stabilizes at that level. Once the initial criterion is reached, large incentives, such as monetary reward, are delivered and a new, more stringent criterion is established. Treatment then continues until a stable response rate is demonstrated at the new criterion level, incentives are delivered and the criterion is again changed. The remainder of the phase progresses in a step-like manner with each criterion adjustment more closely approximating a terminal level and it concludes when responding stabilizes at that level.

Experimental control is demonstrated with the changing-criterion design when the change in the target behavior closely corresponds to and stabilizes at each new criterion level. Stable responding at each criterion level provides a "baseline" for successive treatment phases and the co-occurrence of change in the behavior and shift in criterion levels during each treatment phase provides within-subject replication of the experimental effect. Thus, control elements previously discussed for the multiple-baseline design, stable base rate and replication, are also evident in the changing-criterion design.

Phase Length, Magnitude, and Number of Criterion Changes

The changing-criterion design has seldom been reported in the applied literature and appropriate implementation of this strategy depends, therefore, on logical rather than proven procedural considerations. Hartmann and Hall (1976) have, however, suggested that three design factors; length of experimental phases, magnitude, and number of criterion changes are crucial aspects of the changing-criterion design and each of these factors will be briefly examined.

The most important consideration in establishing the length of baseline and treatment phases of a changing-criterion study is that the phases must be long enough to demonstrate that behavioral changes are not due to factors extraneous to treatment. Kazdin (1977b; 1980) notes that behavioral change associated with the changing-criterion design is unidirectional and increases or decreases in behavior may, therefore, be due to nontreatment variables. That is, the changing-criterion design basically conforms to an A-B design with a criterion interrupted treatment phase. Recognizing this, Hartmann and Hall (1976) suggested that investigators vary the length of treatment phases whenever possible, or, if phases are the same length, they ". . .should be preceded by a baseline phase longer than each of the separate treatment phases" (p. 530). These precautions may avoid criterion changes that parallel any "naturally" occurring increases or decreases in subject responses. These authors also indicate that longer baseline and treatment phases may be needed to establish a stable rate of responding for variable behaviors.

The magnitude of criterion changes will also be influenced by variability of subject responses, and larger criterion changes may be necessary to demonstrate treatment effects for highly variable target behaviors. Additional considerations relevant to establishing the magnitude of criterion changes include total amount of change desired and the type of behavior being investigated. For example, the magnitude should be small enough to permit a sufficient number of criterion changes for replications of the treatment effect. Finally, Hall and Fox (1977) have proposed using the mean baseline performance as a guideline for establishing an initial criterion level. Using the average baseline performance as a guideline may ensure that the established level is within the subject's capabilities.

The appropriate number of treatment phases or criterion changes in a changing-criterion study can only be determined on a study-by-study basis. Essentially, the investigator must decide how many replications are sufficient to demonstrate experimental control. Although Hartmann and Hall (1976) state that two criterion changes may be adequate when change in subject behavior closely parallels the changing criterion, more replications are recommended. The changing-criterion design may not be as powerful as the reversal and multiple-baseline designs (Kazdin, 1977b and c, 1980) and additional changes in criterion will strengthen the conclusions that can be made when this design is employed. In addition, replication across subjects is necessary to demonstrate unequivocal treatment results when the changing-criterion design is used. The following hypothetical example demonstrates these and other important aspects of the changing-criterion design.

The subject of this study is a 10-year-old boy with small bilateral vocal nodules at the junction of the anterior and middle third of the vocal folds who had exhibited a moderate degree of hoarseness in all speaking situations for several weeks before the initiation of the study. Although preexperimental examination did not reveal any vocal misuses that might have contributed to his nodules and voice quality problem, his parents and teacher reported that he was frequently observed "yelling and screaming" during school recess periods in the gymnasium and at the playground near his home. It was decided, therefore, that the initial emphasis in treatment would be to reduce the vocally abusive behaviors exhibited during play periods, because vocal abuse may result in nodules and voice quality problems (Brodnitz, 1971). Before the study the child was observed during school recess and on the playground to determine the exact nature of the abusive behaviors so that they could be targeted for reduction. Furthermore, through parental interview it was determined that the subject regularly attended a weekend swim group with his father and other neighborhood parents and children. The parents reported that the boy enjoyed this weekend outing and they agreed that attendance at the weekly sessions might provide a strong contingency that could be used in an abuse-reduction program.

The experimental phases of this changing-criterion study were as follows. During baseline, independent examiners observed and recorded vocal abuse during 1-hour daily school recess activities across five consecutive school days. The treatment phase began at the completion of baseline measurement and the goal of treatment was to reduce the number of vocal abuses exhibited during the daily recess sessions in the gymnasium. The treatment package included self monitoring of vocal abuses during recess periods and daily "points" given for accurate self-monitoring and meeting preestablished criterion levels for vocal abuses. In addition, an accummulation of a specified number of points was required for the boy to attend the weekly swim session.

During each baseline session the subject produced approximately 25 vocal abuses. The initial criterion level was, therefore, set at 20 or fewer abuses per session plus 85% or greater agreement with the experimenter on the number of self recorded abuses. Performance had to be stabilized at this level for three consecutive sessions before the criterion was made more stringent. If the boy met this criterion, he was allowed to attend the weekend recreational session with his father. Otherwise, he was not allowed to go to the swim session. During the remainder of the treatment phase the criterion was changed by requiring the boy to produce five fewer abuses in each successive step in the program. The self-monitoring and stability criteria remained unchanged throughout the treatment phase and the weekend recreational contingency also remained in effect.

The results of this hypothetical study are presented in Figure 35. Note that a stable rate of responding was obtained during the baseline phase of the investigation. In addition, once treatment was initiated reductions in the number of vocal abuses closely correspond to changes in the criterion level. Furthermore, after each criterion level was met the target behavior stabilized at that level until a new criterion was established. In essence, the data reveal four replications of the treatment effect, one at each criterion level, and they provide a convincing demonstration of a functional relationship between intervention and the reduction in vocally abusive behaviors.

For the sake of simplicity, little has been said about the subject's hoarseness, despite the fact that this would have been a primary concern in a study of this nature. Had this been a true-to-life example, data also would have been obtained on the effect of treatment on the child's voice quality so that the investigator could determine if the vocal abuses had indeed been responsible for the voice problem. Given this qualification, let us now turn our attention to other practical aspects of the changing-criterion design.

Additional Considerations

Although the changing-criterion design may not be as powerful as the reversal or multiple-baseline designs (Kazdin, 1977b; 1980), slight modifications in the design add believability to obtained results. For example, a brief reversal phase may be incorporated by reverting to a previous criterion level (Hall and Fox, 1977). Returning to our example, a reversal might have been implemented after the subject reached the criterion of ten or fewer vocal abuses (Figure 35). Had this been attempted, the criterion could have been returned to the previously obtained level of fifteen abuses rather than making the criterion more stringent by changing it to five or fewer abuses per session. Similarly, a removal of all experimental contingencies might have been undertaken to determine if this would affect the subject's rate of responding. In either case, a return toward baseline level responding would have provided

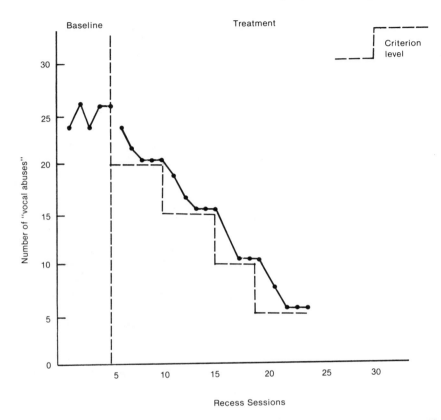

Figure 35. Hypothetical data depicting the number of "vocal abuses" produced by a 10-year-old boy with vocal nodules during daily school recess sessions.

additional evidence of experimental control. Another procedure for strengthening the changing-criterion design which has been proposed by Hartmann and Hall (1976) is to lengthen one or more treatment phases. If the behavior change remains at a given criterion level when a treatment phase is lengthened, additional evidence is provided that the change is related to the criterion level.

As we have noted, the changing-criterion design is most appropriate for examining behaviors acquired gradually (Hall and Fox, 1977). Behaviors acquired rapidly are not likely to parallel frequent criterion changes or stabilize at a given level long enough to demonstrate experimental control. As a result, this design may not be appropriate for studying behaviors that exhibit periods of accelerated acquisition such as articulation or auditory discrimination. This design does, however, have several advantages over other single-subject research designs. It does not require an investigator to extinguish or reverse behavior as withdrawal or reversal designs do, and only one behavior is selected for treatment rather than the two or more required to carry out a multiple-baseline study (Hartmann and Hall, 1976). Possible confounding due to order effects and the need to counterbalance treatment order are also avoided when a single behavior is targeted for treatment.

A final advantage of the changing-criterion design is that it is well suited for examining generalization across settings, people, and time. Recall that the child in our example had exhibited vocally abusive behaviors during school recess periods and on the playground near his home. Although intervention was only undertaken during school recess periods, the study could have been expanded by monitoring generalization of reductions in vocal abuses for specified times at the playground. The child's voice problem might have persisted after successful elimination of "screaming and yelling" during recess, if there was not a concomitant reduction of abuses at the playground, swimming pool, and so on. If the effects of training did not generalize, programming could be initiated in these settings. Similar modifications of this study could be devised to evaluate generalization to individuals outside of the school setting and to assess maintenance of treatment gains.

The changing-criterion design is not the only variation of the multiple-baseline design that is well suited for examining generalization. A second modification of the multiple-baseline design that can be adopted for studying generalization issues, the multiple-probe design, is examined in the following section.

MULTIPLE-PROBE DESIGN

Training a terminal behavior may involve the chaining of smaller components of that behavior and successive steps in the chaining sequence may be impossible or extremely difficult without the acquisition of earlier steps in the sequence. For example, before reaching the terminal behavior of conversational esophageal speech production, a laryngectomized individual must first be trained to phonate consistently on command and produce selected words and phrases. Moreover, criterion level performance for voicing and single-word production would be considered necessary prerequisites to achieving the terminal goal of conversational speech. Yet, despite our assumptions about presumed relationships between steps in a chaining sequence, we cannot be sure that the steps within a sequence are as independent as they seem. Some clients or subjects may generalize their newly acquired behaviors rapidly and they need little or no training at a given step in a treatment hierarchy. On the other hand, there are instances in which con-

tinuous probing of later behaviors in a training sequence would be inefficient, because the interdependence between steps in the chain are either predictable or well established. One would not, for example, spend considerable
time probing phrases or sentence-level esophageal speech production for a
subject who did not phonate consistently or for a sufficient duration. Similarly, it may be inefficient to take continuous baseline data over extended
periods of time for untreated behaviors in a multiple-baseline study if there
is strong evidence that the behaviors are stable and not likely to change.
A balance must be reached between the amount of information needed
to demonstrate experimental control and the practical aspects of a given
study. One design that may be used to reach this balance is the multiple-
probe design.

The multiple-probe design is a practical alternative to the multiple-
baseline design for investigations of chained behaviors or steps in a successive
approximation sequence and it also provides an alternative to multiple-
baseline studies requiring long or continuous baseline measurements
(Horner and Baer, 1978). This design is actually a combination of a multiple-
baseline design and probe procedures.[1] According to Horner and Baer (1978)
there are three primary features of the multiple-probe technique, including:
1) an initial probe of every step in a chain or successive approximation, 2) a
probe of each step in the treatment sequence after criterion is achieved on any
step, and 3) a series of probes or "true baselines" immediately before the initiation of training on any given step in the sequence. The series of probes
conducted before intervention on any step in training are considered "true
baselines" because it is presumed that later steps cannot be performed until
earlier steps have been acquired. Thus, only probes following the completion
of all prerequisite steps and immediately before intervention are considered a
true measure of the subject's ability to perform a given step. Horner and Baer
(1978) recommend that true baselines be increased by one or more additional
probes for each successive step in the training sequence. Thus, the "true
baseline" preceding the second step in a training program would include two
or more probes and the baseline before intervention for the third step would
include at least three probes. The exact nature of the probes, in terms of the
number of trials given and stimulus conditions for testing, are dependent
upon the behaviors being investigated and practical considerations such as
the amount of time available for testing.

The multiple-probe design has only recently been reported and there
are, therefore, few examples of this design in the communicative disorders

---

[1]For the purposes of the discussion a probe will be considered an intermittent assessment of
selected target behaviors under nontreatment conditions. Responses to probe items are not
generally consequated and probes are often used to assess the generalization of training.

literature. Roodenburg and Smeets (1980) reported a study, however, that can be used to demonstrate the multiple-probe technique. The purpose of this study was to train a mentally retarded quadriplegic individual to use an electronic communication board, and there were four steps in the training procedure. First, the subject was trained to operate a reset key that illuminated a light on the display panel of the communication board and signaled the end of a communicative attempt. The second and third steps in the program involved operation of vertical and horizontal direction keys. These keys controlled the direction that a signal light traveled while the board was in operation. For example, the horizontal key illuminated a light beneath a square on the display panel to the right of the reset square. The final training step required the subject to press an alarm key, which set off a loud signal to alert a listener to attend to the display panel. Criterion performance at each training level was based on successful completion of the step being trained as well as all previous steps. Thus, to complete successfully the final phase of training, the subject had to carry out all three previous steps in addition to operating the alarm key on each trial of this phase.

The design of this study involved probing the subject's performance on the terminal (step 4) behavior before training on each step in the program. Although this study did not use a multiple-probe design, the multiple-probe technique could have been employed with the following modifications as shown in Figure 36. Initially, a separate probe would have been obtained for each step in the program and, assuming that the subject was unable to produce the required behaviors, treatment would have been implemented to teach the subject to operate the reset key (step 1). Once criterion was achieved for the first step, a probe would have been administered to evaluate performance on the three remaining steps. In addition, a second probe would have been necessary for the second step, operation of the vertical direction key, in order to establish a true baseline for this step. Treatment would then have been initiated on this behavior until the criterion level was met. At that point, performance on the third and fourth step would again be probed and two additional probes of step three, operation of horizontal direction key, would be necessary to establish a true baseline for this step. Finally, upon reaching criterion for manipulation of the horizontal key, four successive probes would be administered to establish a baseline for operating the alerting alarm and training would begin on this final step. The graphic display of these hypothetical data is presented in Figure 36.

Several aspects of the data are noteworthy. First, notice that the data display for the multiple-probe design closely resembles the graphic display used for multiple-baseline studies. This is not, of course, coincidental. Probes and true baselines along the abscissa can be examined, just as the baseline phase of a multiple-baseline study would be, to determine if the

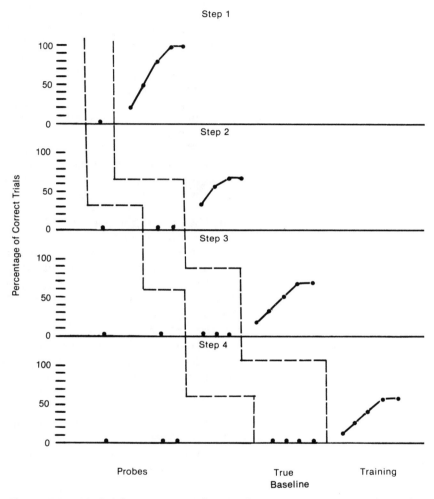

Figure 36. Hypothetical data. Percentage of correct trials across a 4–step program designed to teach a retarded quadriplegic subject how to operate an electronic language board (after Roodenberg and Smeets, 1980).

behaviors remained stable until intervention was initiated at each step in the training sequence. Examination of the graph reveals that the probe and true baseline data remained unchanged, essentially at the 0% correct level, until treatment was initiated. In addition, examination of the training data reveals that performance at each step in the program improved only after treatment. Based on these hypothetical data, one might conclude that the treatment program was responsible for improvements noted in the use of the communication board. As this brief example demonstrates, the multiple-probe design can provide a means of efficiently evaluating the steps in a training program. Experimental control can be demonstrated with this design, despite the fact that less baseline data are available, as long as the pretreated probe and true baseline data are stable and a consistent treatment effect is shown. Let us now examine a second example of the multiple-probe design and consider its use as an alternative to the continuous data collection procedures employed in multiple-baseline designs.

Horner and Baer (1978) have noted that continuous baseline testing of untreated behaviors in a multiple-baseline design may be reactive and / or impractical. That is, extended baselines can result in "extinction, boredom, and fatigue, or other effects" (Horner and Baer, 1978, p. 174). In addition, continuous baseline measurement may not be necessary when there is a strong a priori assumption that a stable base rate will be obtained. This may be the case, for example, for behaviors that are not expected to change without treatment. Finally, Horner and Baer also suggest that intermittent baseline observations may approximate the level of accuracy obtained through continuous testing, and the multiple-probe technique may, therefore, be used as an alternative to the session-by-session measurement used in multiple-baseline designs. The following example demonstrates the use of a multiple-probe procedure during baseline testing.

Tucker and Berry (1980) examined the effectiveness of a training program designed to teach three severely handicapped children to put on their hearing aids. There were ten components to the training program and multiple steps within each component. Although there were slight individual variations in the program, each subject was trained on three "universal" components. Steps within these components required the subjects to obtain an aid from its container, fasten the aid to a harness or T-shirt pocket, turn the aid on, and adjust the gain (loudness) control. Additional training components included putting on the hearing aid harness or T-shirt, and inserting an earmold or putting on a bone-conduction head band.

During the treatment phase of this investigation, steps in the program were sequentially trained through a graded series of prompts that ranged from "No Help" to "Physical Guidance and Assistance." Prompts were given after each incorrect response and praise was provided after each step in the chain was successfully completed.

The dependent variable in this investigation was the percentage of training steps completed in each session without experimenter assistance. The effect of treatment on the dependent measure was evaluated by using a modified multiple-baseline design across subjects. Multiple-probe sessions replaced continuous testing during the initial portion of the baseline phase.

Generalization to a classroom and residential living environment was intermittently probed throughout the investigation. The results of this study are shown in Figure 37.

Of particular interest to this discussion is the baseline, multiple-probe data depicted for Randy and Steve. Note that for these subjects true baselines were not begun until sessions 14 and 31, respectively, and occasional probes replaced continuous measurement during early baseline sessions. Both subjects performed at a relatively low rate of responding on these probes and this level approximated the level produced during true baseline testing. This, in combination with stable true baseline performance, indicates that continuous measurement during the early baseline phase might have resulted in a response pattern similar to that obtained during the true baseline phase.

Visual inspection of the data led the authors to conclude that the treatment program was successful in training Randy and Steve to put on their

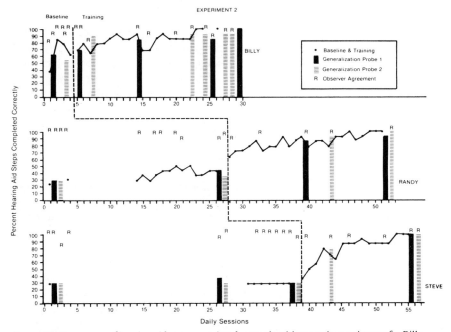

Figure 37. Percentage of hearing aid steps completed correctly without trainer assistance for Billy, Randy, and Steve. The *crosshatched bars* represent probe performance in the education classroom; the *solid bars* represent probe performance in the residential areas. The *connected dots* represent continuous consecutive sessions of either baseline or training in the training area; *unconnected dots* represent periodic consecutive baseline sessions. Probe data are temporally superimposed over the training area data. The *R* represents the level of reliability agreement for a given session. (From Tucker and Berry, 1980, p. 73. Copyright by Society for the Experimental Analysis of Behavior, Inc. Reproduced by permission).

hearing aids. The effect of the training on the third subject's performance could not be determined because of his high and variable rate of responding during baseline. Finally, a close correspondence was noted between the subject's performance in the training setting and performance in the two generalization settings.

This study demonstrates the feasibility of substituting intermittent probing for continuous testing during the baseline phase of a multiple-baseline study. Although this investigation used a modified multiple-baseline design across subjects, the use of the multiple-probe technique appears equally applicable to investigations using multiple-baseline designs across behaviors or settings.

Additional Considerations

The multiple-probe design is a cost-effective alternative to the multiple-baseline design (Murphy and Bryan, 1980). It reduces the amount of time spent on scheduling and conducting baseline sessions when it is used to replace continuous baseline measurement and it facilitates efficient treatment programming when used to investigate the steps in a training sequence. The systematic probing of each step in a training sequence fosters efficient treatment programming by revealing the presence and extent of generalization across training steps (Horner and Baer, 1978). Training on the initial steps of a sequence may facilitate partial or complete performance of later steps and thereby reduce the amount of training required and/or eliminate the need to train one or more steps in a program.

Although the multiple-probe technique is generally an efficient design strategy, it may prove impractical for examining treatment programs that have a large number of training steps. Horner and Baer (1978), for example, note that when the multiple-probe design is employed to examine a ten–step training program, the final step in the program is preceded by nine probe and ten true baseline sessions. Because the practicality of such a large number of probes is questionable, they suggest dividing large programs into smaller segments and then separately applying the probe technique to the steps within each segment in order to limit the number of probes administered. An unfortunate result of this approach, however, is the loss of valuable information about the facilitative effects of training. That is, when large programs are divided into smaller segments examined separately, initial probes are not obtained on later steps and any generalization to later steps as a result of earlier training cannot be detected. For example, if a ten–step program was divided into two segments, initial probes would only be obtained on the first five steps and performance on steps 6 through 10 would not be probed until criterion was met for the fifth training step. As a result, one could not determine if high-level performance on later steps in the program occurred after training on the first five steps, or, if a high level would also have been obtained on initial, pretraining probes. The second alternative would be particularly plausible when an investigator is examining a training sequence for which there is no previous literature to support the component steps or order of a training sequence.

The limitations of Horner and Baer's (1978) suggestions for examining training programs having a large number of training steps can be circumvented by adopting a sequential probe procedure that could be implemented as follows. First, an initial baseline probe would be obtained on all steps in a program. Subsequently, additional probes would be obtained on a predetermined number of steps in the program (perhaps three) after criterion was met on any given step. Finally, true baselines could be adjusted to a reasonable maximum number according to the exigencies of a given study. In a ten-step sequence, for example, all steps would be probed during the initial baseline probe session. After this, training would be implemented on the first step until the criterion was met. At that point, an additional probe would be obtained on steps 2 through 4 and a true baseline would also be obtained on step 2. Assuming that performance had not appreciably changed on step 2, training would be implemented on this step until the criterion was met. Probes would then be obtained on steps 3 through 5 of the program. A true baseline and training on step 3 would follow. This sequence would then be repeated until the criterion was met on the tenth training step. Depending on the exact nature of the study, the number of true baseline probes obtained for any step in the program might not be allowed to exceed five. Although arbitrary, this would provide a sufficient demonstration of true baseline stability without being impractical. The number of true baseline probes could, of course, be varied as an additional control measure.

The sequential probe technique provides initial probe data on each step in a training program so that performance change on later steps in the program can be evaluated. In addition, the sequence of probes administered after a criterion is met on any step in the program provides more and earlier data on later training steps than would be provided by segmenting a program into smaller parts. Finally, the procedure offers a compromise between the data loss associated with dividing large programs and the excessive probing required to obtain continuous data on each step of a training sequence.

Precautionary measures are necessary to avoid compromising the results of multiple-probe studies. For example, guidelines do not currently exist for determining the ideal number of baseline probes needed to provide a convincing demonstration of stability when multiple probes replace continuous-baseline testing. Horner and Baer's (1978) multiple-probing procedures for evaluating steps in a training sequence should be incorporated when the multiple-probe technique replaces session-by-session baseline measurement.

At a minimum, an initial baseline probe and a true baseline should be obtained (see Tucker and Berry, 1980).

Subtle control problems can also arise when the multiple-probe design is used to evaluate the steps in a training program. In discussing the need for a true baseline, Horner and Baer (1978, p. 192) note that successive steps in a program are "assumed to be impossible or unlikely" until previous steps in the chain are acquired. It should be cautioned, however, this design may not be appropriate for studying program steps that are truly interdependent. That is, if sequential steps in a training sequence cannot be performed before criterion is met on preceding steps, a zero baseline is guaranteed on later steps in the sequence. Although the low level of responding on the later steps will present the appearance of a stable base rate and experimental control, the use of interdependent behaviors ensures that there is no opportunity for change in the untreated behaviors. As a result, extraneous variables that might affect experimental results are not likely to be detected because a "loss of baseline" is not possible.

Horner and Baer (1978) state that "the multiple-probe technique avoids the collection of a continuous series of ritualistic, pro forma zero baseline points when performance of any component of a chain of behaviors or a successive-approximation sequence is impossible or very unlikely before acquisition of its preceding component" (p. 195). Although the design does avoid unnecessary probing of behaviors that are not expected to change, it does not provide a convincing means of experimental control when the functional relationship between a treatment variable and performance on steps in a training sequence is examined, even though this is one of the major purposes of the multiple-probe procedure. Analysis of interdependent training steps is equivalent to a series of A-B studies on each of several independent behaviors and the limitation of this quasi-experimental approach must be considered when the multiple-probe design is used in this manner. Totally interdependent baseline behaviors can only provide the appearance of experimental control and should not be studied with the multiple-probe design.

The multiple-probe design has not yet been used extensively by applied researchers. Additional investigations are needed to demonstrate which communicative disorders treatment programs can be investigated with this type of treatment design. The design's usefulness as an alternative to continuous baseline measurement has been established, but additional information is needed regarding its appropriateness for evaluating the steps in training sequences.

The multiple-probe design shares both the advantages and limitations of the multiple-baseline design. Thus, similar but independent behaviors must be chosen for study in order to avoid a "loss of baseline" and experimental control. Alternately, reversal of behavior change is not necessary for demonstrating experimental control and the design may, therefore, be particularly useful in applied settings in which staff resistance to reversal or withdrawal procedures is expected. As previously noted, the multiple-probe design avoids problems of extinction, fatigue, and distraction that can occur as a result of continuous-baseline testing. Furthermore, it is a potentially efficient means of evaluating the effects of training on sequential steps in a treatment program for behaviors that are not totally interdependent. As such, it is the only formalized within-case experimental design that includes a procedure for examining generalization across steps in a training program. Other types of generalization, for example, generalization across settings, may also be assessed with this design. The topic of generalization probe procedures is further considered in the section that follows.

GENERALIZATION PROBE PROCEDURES

Applied investigators of communicative disorders have been primarily concerned with the acquisition of speech and language behaviors and relatively few studies have examined issues relating to generalization. Moreover, reviews of the available literature indicates that trained speech and language behaviors do not automatically generalize to conditions or settings outside the training environment (Garcia and DeHaven, 1974; Harris, 1975) despite the commonly held assumption that generalization occurs whenever treatment is successful (Marholin, Siegel, and Phillips, 1976). Thus, investigative efforts are needed to determine the nature and extent of the generalization of trained communicative behaviors and to isolate factors that may facilitate generative responding. As Guess, Keogh, and Sailor (1978) note, ''a new language user's competence is determined primarily through a demonstrated ability to generalize appropriately. Likewise, the efficiency of the intervention process itself must be judged by how well it teaches generalized language use'' (p. 376).

Before discussing experimental designs and probe procedures that have been used to investigate generalization, it may be beneficial to consider briefly several factors relating to this issue. Stokes and Baer (1977) reviewed several hundred experimental investigations of generalization in an attempt to summarize this literature and describe trends that might be used to develop a technology of generalization. They defined generalization as ''the occurrence of relevant behavior under different non-training conditions (i.e., across subjects, settings, people, behaviors, and/or time) without the scheduling of the same events in those conditions as had been scheduled in the training conditions'' (p. 350). A recurring theme throughout this review is the belief that applied researchers have viewed generalization as a natural outcome of the treatment process. That is, it has not been a phenomenon that has been actively pursued, or for which specific techniques have been developed. Rather, generalization has been viewed passively. Failure to obtain generalized responding has been considered a natural result of experimental techniques that resulted in stringent control over stimuli and responses. Thus, training techniques are often designed to facilitate discrimination between conditions that set the occasion for responding and those that do not. As a result of this emphasis on discrimination training procedures, learning is often situation specific and behaviors learned under highly discriminable conditions may not generalize to other settings or people or across time (Marholin et al., 1976).

The results of the Stokes and Baer (1977) review support their contention that applied investigators have viewed generalization as a passive phenomenon. Nearly half of the studies examined for this extensive review were classified as *Train and Hope* investigations. That is, generalization was probed for and reported when it occurred, but procedures that might have facilitated carry-over were not examined and no attempt was made to improve responding in those instances in which generalization did not occur. Further evidence that investigators have not attempted to develop a technology of generalization has also been provided by Hayes, Rincover, and Solnick (1980). After reviewing studies reported during the first decade of publication of the *Journal of Applied Behavior Analysis,* these authors found a disturbing trend in the literature. They note that, despite an increase in the number of investigations that examined the maintenance of treatment effects, investigations of generalization across settings, stimuli, and untrained responses seem to be decreasing in numbers. Based on the results of these reviews it would seem that Baer, Wolf, and Risley's (1968) admonition that ". . . generalization should be programmed, rather than expected or lamented" (p. 97) has not been taken seriously. Although authors of comprehensive reviews of the applied generalization literature have provided suggestions for facilitating generalization (Wildman and Wildman, 1975; Marholin et al., 1976; Stokes and Baer, 1977; Guess, Keogh, and Sailor, 1978), the usefulness of these suggestions has not been demonstrated experimentally. Investigators of communicative disorders and other applied problems have not explored factors that may result in generalized responding for specified subjects and training conditions, and obtaining such information may present "one of the foremost challenges" (Hayes et al., 1980) to developing efficacious treatment programs.

Factors that facilitate generative responding have seldom been investigated in the applied literature, despite the fact that generative responding is the ultimate aim of most training programs (Spradlin, Karlan, and Wetherby, 1976). Often, acquisition data are discussed in depth, whereas generalization data are treated descriptively as an added point of interest, although this trend appears to be changing (Kearns and Salmon, in press; Solomon, 1981; Elbert and McReynolds, 1978). Generative responding is seldom the primary dependent variable in applied communicative disorders research.

Given the absence of objective information in this area and the critical nature of the topic of generalization, this discussion focuses on generalization probe procedures employed in within-subject experimental designs. Probe techniques are discussed in conjunction with their underlying rationale for generalization across three categories: behavior, situation, and time. These categories are not all inclusive; they are, however, especially relevant to clinical intervention research (O'Leary and Drabman, 1971; Wahler, Berland, and Coe, 1979).

Generalization Across Behaviors

Of the three classes of generalization to be examined, behavior analysts have investigated transfer from trained to untrained behaviors most extensively. Furthermore, investigators have been more successful in demonstrating generalization across behaviors than they have been in demonstrating generalization across situations or time. We will begin our consideration of generalization across behaviors with a brief description of response classes, an important concept underlying this area of research.

The notion of functional or generative response classes has been an integral aspect of behavioral accounts of language acquisition (Salzinger, 1967). In addition, it has been used to explain the occurrence of generative responding that has resulted from language treatment based on imitation and differential reinforcement training procedures (Guess and Baer, 1973). Early training studies of the acquisition of grammatical morphemes, for example, demonstrated that training a sufficient number of target responses often results in generalized responding to untrained exemplars of that same class of behaviors (Sailor, 1971; Baer and Guess, 1971; Guess and Baer, 1973). These findings have been replicated for sentence (Wheeler and Sulzer, 1970; Lutzker and Sherman, 1974; Clark and Sherman, 1975) and conversational responding (Garcia, 1974). Language responses are, it seems, organized into a variety of functional classes, and training a subset of responses within a class will result in generalized responding to other members of that class of behaviors. Stated otherwise, when trained and untrained behaviors co-vary, the responses are viewed as belonging to the same functional or generative response class. In this respect, generalization across behaviors is a primary criterion for determining the interrelationship among linguistic behaviors, and generalization probe procedures provide the mechanism for assessing these functional relationships.

In the following section we examine probe procedures frequently used to assess generalization across behaviors. The notion of "procedural contrast" is also discussed, because the rationale for the probe techniques is inextricably linked to this phenomenon.

Procedural Contrast and Generalization Probe Procedures

An essential consideration in designing a study to investigate generalization is the procedural contrast between reinforced training items and unreinforced probe items. Cuvo (1979) has discussed the problem of procedural contrast as it relates to multiple-baseline designs. He notes that training procedures employed in most treatment studies include combining specific discriminative stimuli, feedback, and reinforcement in an attempt to alter the rate of responding. Alternately, feedback and contingent reinforcement are not generally provided during testing or probing conditions. Consequently, training and probing phases of an investigation may be easily discriminated and subjects may not respond or generalize to nonreinforced probes. In addition, when generative responding does occur to probe items, it may be readily extinguished because of the lack of contingent feedback and consequation. Communicative disorders investigators should, therefore, use generalization probe procedures that minimize procedural contrast between training and probing conditions.

Perhaps the most common method employed to reduce the deleterious effects of procedural contrast is to intermix reinforced training items and generalization items during generalization probe sessions. Many of the previously cited response class studies employed this technique to examine generalization across trained language behaviors. Baer and Guess (1971), for example, interspersed probe and training trials during their examination of receptive training of adjective suffixes in mentally retarded subjects. A multiple-baseline design across behaviors was employed and receptive understanding of comparative (e.g., small_er_) and superlative (e.g., small_est_) grammatical markers was investigated. The probing procedures employed in this study were as follows.

During training phases a variable-ratio 3 (VR3) reinforcement schedule was established so that unreinforced probes could be interspersed with training items. Because, on the average, every third correct response is consequated using this schedule, probe items were substituted for training items on trials for which reinforcement was not available. Thus, although correct responses to training items were consequated on the variable ratio schedule, nonreinforced probe items were also simultaneously administered. Several types of probes were obtained in this manner. For example, probes of un-trained exemplars of the comparative and probes of the untrained superlative constructions were administered during comparative training. The results of this study demonstrated that receptive training on comparative or superlative suffixes resulted in generative responding to novel combinations of the trained constructions. Although the probing procedure employed in this study was not directly compared with alternate procedures, interspersing training and probe items may have minimized procedural contrast and facilitated generative responding.

Interspersing training and probe items to minimize procedural contrast has become a frequent practice in the applied communicative disorders literature. Often, separate probes are conducted to assess generalization to untrained but similar behaviors once an item or a subset of items within a training set have been trained to criterion (Lutzker and Sherman, 1974; Frisch and Schumaker, 1974; Schreibman and Carr, 1978; Hegde and Gierut, 1979). Hegde (1980), for example, incorporated separate interspersed probe sessions into his study of auxiliary and copula verb generalization. Two language-delayed children who omitted the present tense auxiliary and copular verb *is* served as subjects in this study. Using an A-B-A-B reversal design, one subject was trained, reversed, and retrained on verbal production of the present tense auxiliary and the second subject underwent the same experimental sequence for the copula form. The dependent variable was verbal production of untrained exemplars of the auxiliary or copular verb. Generalization to the untrained construction (i.e., copula for S_1 and auxiliary for S_2) was probed throughout each phase of the investigation and the generalization probe procedures were as follows. Six sentences were targeted for auxiliary or copula training and sixty items were used to assess generalization. Half of the generalization items were auxiliary sentences and the remaining half were copula sentences. Target sentence items were individually trained and a probe was conducted to evaluate generalization after criterion was met on two sentences. Both auxiliary and copula items were presented during probe sessions and a fixed-ratio 2 (FR2) schedule of reinforcement was implemented so that training and generalization items could be intermixed. Because reinforcement is available after every other correct response on an FR2 schedule, nonreinforced probe items were alternated with reinforced training items. When a specified generalization criterion was not met on the first probe, two additional items were trained and a second probe was conducted. Training and probing continued in this manner until criterion was finally met. The results of this study demonstrated generalization to untrained exemplars of the trained auxiliary and copula construction for subjects 1 and 2, respectively. In addition, the first subject generalized *is* when responding to copula items, despite having only been trained on auxiliary sentences. Similarly, copula training was sufficient to obtain generative auxiliary responding for the second subject.

The previous examples demonstrate one procedure for making training and probe conditions less discriminable and minimizing the effects of procedural contrast. Alternate procedures, such as using noncontingent reinforcement during probe conditions, may also be employed for this purpose. Garcia (1974) employed this technique in a study of acquisition and generalization of a conversational speech form with two retarded subjects. Three separate short sentences were individually trained, and then chained with an examiner's verbalization to form a short conversational unit. Generalization was probed to untrained stimuli and examiners during "general" and "intermixed" probe sessions. Intermixed probe procedures were previously described and will not be further considered. During "general" probe sessions, picture stimuli and specified verbal responses were presented in an attempt to elicit a target conversational sequence. The delivery of noncontingent reinforcement was described as follows. "Reinforcement during these sessions was provided on the average of once each minute, with the stipulation that reinforcement occur between probe trials and at least 10 seconds after any verbal response emitted by the subject" (Garcia, 1974, p. 140).

The results of this study indicated that both subjects acquired the conversational speech chain but generalization across examiners was negligible when general probe sessions were conducted. Generalization of the trained verbal response to untrained stimuli and to an examiner was obtained after intermixed probe sessions were conducted. Although the authors apparently felt that the intermixing procedure facilitated generative responding, effects of the two probe techniques are difficult to separate. The probes were administered in a set sequence and the influence of the order of presentation may have been an important determinant of the results.

Although additional research is needed to examine the variety of generalization probe procedures available, it would appear that the intermixing technique and use of noncontingent reinforcement during probe sessions may circumvent the deleterious effects of procedural contrast. Although these techniques were discussed within the context of generalization across behaviors, they may also be useful for examining other forms of generalization. In the following section we begin exploring additional considerations in generalization probing, particularly as they relate to generalization across situations.

Generalization Across Situations

Applied communicative disorders research is frequently conducted in clinical or laboratory environments because a degree of experimental control can be obtained that is difficult to achieve in the natural environment. Ironically, the ultimate test of our therapeutic techniques is whether they have a meaningful and lasting impact within the home, school, and other daily living settings and generality of laboratory data to these environments is open to question. It may, of course, be necessary to build the data base needed to treat complex communicative impairments in well-controlled environments before assessing the generality to other situations. Too often, however, generality to other situations is simply never examined. Therefore, the purpose of this discussion is to examine issues and procedures relevant to probing generalization of trained behaviors to nontraining situations.

In the previous discussion we alluded to the need to minimize procedural contrast when probing for generalization across behaviors. An implicit assumption of this suggestion was that generalization and discrimination are, to a certain extent, reciprocally related, and maintaining similarities between training and probing conditions may reduce the degree of discriminability between conditions and facilitate generative responding. Although our discussion of procedural contrast emphasized the need to minimize differences between the consequent events available during training and probing, it is equally important to maintain similar settings and other discriminative stimuli in training and testing conditions. In short, an important procedural consideration in examining generalization across situations is that maximizing similarities between treatment and probe settings may enhance the probability of obtaining generalization (Stokes and Baer, 1977; Guess et al., 1978). Logically, the opposite may also be true. Increasing the differences between training and generalization probe conditions would be expected to reduce the probability of obtaining generalization across situations.

The cumulative results of studies that have examined the generalization of trained spontaneous communicative behaviors across examiners or settings indicate that transfer is often limited unless specific procedures are implemented to facilitate generative responding (Johnston and Johnston, 1972; Garcia, 1974; Jackson and Wallace, 1974; Murdock, Garcia, and Hardman, 1977; Handelman, 1981). It is noteworthy that several variables are altered simultaneously in studies of generalization across situations and it is therefore impossible to determine which factor or combination of factors influenced obtained results. Murdock, Garcia, and Hardman (1977), for example, evaluated generalization of the effects of articulation training with retarded subjects. A multiple-baseline design across behaviors (misarticulated words) was employed in this study. Initially, the first experimenter trained a selected word in setting 1 and probed generalization to four other settings (2–5) and examiners. Training was initiated in settings 2 through 4 if a preselected generalization criterion was not met in these situations. No training was ever conducted in the fifth setting. The remaining target words were sequentially trained after the first word had sufficiently generalized to settings 2 through 4 or training had been conducted in each of these settings. The results of this study indicated that generalization of correct production of target words to other settings with other examiners was obtained after additional training was initiated in at least one setting other than the initial treatment setting. In discussing their results Murdock et al. (1977) rightly point out that simultaneous training was conducted by different experimenters in different treatment settings and one or both factors may have been responsible for the generative responding that was obtained. These findings highlight the need to isolate carefully factors that may facilitate generalization across situations. The relative contribution of multiple factors cannot be evaluated when generalization occurs, and when it does not occur, reasons for the negative findings are obscured.

Another convincing reason for isolating variables in studies of generalization is that spontaneous generalization across situations has generally been reported in studies in which a single parameter was varied between training and probing conditions (Carr et al., 1978; Schreibman and Carr, 1978; Welch and Pear, 1980). Carr et al. (1978), for example, investigated the acquisition of expressive sign language in autistic children using a multiple-baseline study across behaviors. Experimenters not associated with training were occasionally introduced into the experimental setting to evaluate generalization across examiners while other aspects of the investigation were held constant. Results indicated that trained expressive sign labels were produced in the presence of new experimenters. As these findings demonstrate, generalization across situations may occur when differences between the testing and training conditions are minimized.

It would appear that a technology of generalization may be developed through investigations of individual factors that purportedly enhance generative responding. In the following discussion of generalization across time, several design options that attempt to isolate such variables are presented.

Generalization Across Time

A treatment program that results in acquisition of a behavior and generalization to similar behaviors and situations will be of limited use if these effects are not maintained over time. Unfortunately, generalization across time is perhaps the least investigated form of transfer. Although practical limitations, such as the time involved in extensive follow-up studies and subject attrition, may make maintenance investigations difficult, it is also likely that the importance and complexity of this issue have simply been overlooked. Moreover, although investigations of generalization across time are being reported with increasing frequency in the applied literature (Hayes et al., 1980), a recent survey of nearly 150 applied studies indicates that only 5% provided follow up data for periods of six months or longer. In the communicative disorders literature, occasional reports of the occurrence of generalization across time are available (Guitar, 1975) but investigation of variables that enhance maintenance have only recently been reported (Ingham, 1975).

In the following discussion we will briefly review Rusch and Kazdin's (1981) suggestions for assessing response maintenance. One additional procedure utilized by Carr et al. (1978) will also be considered. The design options to be discussed, a stimulus-control procedure, sequential withdrawal, partial withdrawal, and partial-sequential withdrawal, do not provide a means of demonstrating experimental control. Rather, these procedures are employed during the maintenance phase of an experiment after one of the previously discussed single-case experimental designs has been used to demonstrate internal validity.

Experimental contingencies are often abruptly removed after training criterion is met, making the training and maintenance phases of an experiment easily discriminable and, perhaps, limiting generalization across time. Furthermore, abrupt withdrawal of contingencies does not permit an assessment of factors, which might encourage maintenance of the newly acquired behavior, and an investigator is not, therefore, in an ideal position for programming maintenance when it does not occur. The following design options may overcome these and other limitations of frequently employed maintenance probe procedures.

Stimulus Control and Sequential-Withdrawal Designs   The sequential-withdrawal design provides a means of evaluating response maintenance when a treatment package with several components is employed (Rusch and Kazdin, 1981). Each component of a treatment package is sequentially removed during consecutive phases of a maintenance period in an attempt to reduce the probability that removal of experimental contingencies will be discriminated. Because this technique is employed after experimental control has been demonstrated, it may be used in conjunction with multiple-baseline, reversal, or any single-subject research strategy.

To date, a sequential withdrawal of components of treatment during a maintenance period has not been reported in the communicative disorders literature. However, Carr et al. (1978) used a stimulus control procedure in their study of the acquisition and generalization of expressive sign labeling in autistic children. Their method provides one means of examining variables that could influence maintenance and it also provides a basis for discussion of the sequential withdrawal of treatment components. A multiple-baseline design across behaviors was used to demonstrate experimental control in this study. A treatment package, consisting of auditory and visual stimuli and prompts, was used to train subjects to produce sign language gestures that corresponded to common food items. During training and testing the experimenter presented a food object or the appropriate sign configuration (visual stimuli) while simultaneously saying the name of an item (auditory stimuli). Physical prompts were initially provided during treatment but they were later faded. Social reinforcement and edibles were provided contingent upon correct sign production. After demonstrating that subjects acquired training signs and their performance generalized across therapists, the investigators initiated a stimulus-control procedure to determine which component of the treatment package was controlling sign production. This post-training assessment consisted of three phases in which only visual, auditory, or speechreading information was available to the subject. In the visual condition an examiner presented a food object, but did not name it, and the subject's ability to produce the appropriate signs was probed. Similarly, in the auditory condition the items were named by the examiner but the food items were not displayed. Finally, in the speechreading condition the examiner inaudibly "mouthed" the name of the items. The results of the stimulus control assessment revealed that three of four subjects responded at a high level in the visual condition but seldom produced appropriate signs in the auditory and speechreading conditions. A fourth subject responded almost perfectly in both the visual and auditory conditions but performed poorly in the speechreading condition.

Returning now to our consideration of the sequential withdrawal procedure, the following modifications in the above study would have demonstrated this technique. After the training phase of the study, one component of the treatment package would have been removed, followed by sequential removal of the remaining components during a follow-up phase to determine which factors would be most likely to maintain the signs. During the first maintenance condition, for example, the auditory stimuli, the names of food items, might have been withdrawn from the probe sessions. Thus, the experimenter would have shown the items to the subjects, and mouthed the names of the items, and subjects would be expected to produce target sign labels. Based on the results of the Carr et al. (1978) study, removal of the auditory input would not be expected to result in a decrease in performance. That is, the visual and speechreading information alone would have been sufficient to maintain accurate responding. In the next maintenance condition the experimenter could decide to withdraw the speechreading input. Thus, only the food items would be presented as stimuli. Again, based on our knowledge of the obtained results, we would anticipate that the visual stimuli alone would be sufficient to control sign production and maintain performance. In general, a sequential withdrawal of the components would have led us to the conclusion that the visual stimuli, rather than the auditory or speechreading stimuli, were likely to facilitate maintenance.

Had the above procedures been implemented, important information would have been available to the investigator. For example, the investigator might believe that the ability to produce expressive sign labels in response to auditory stimuli alone is an important skill that should be trained, and based on the obtained results, remedial procedures to train this skill might have been implemented. However, there are also disadvantages in the sequential withdrawal procedures. For example, Rusch and Kazdin (1981) note that decisions concerning the order in which components are withdrawn or which components will be used to maintain behavior are arbitrary. In the above example the investigators would not have been privy to the results of their stimulus control procedure before starting the sequential withdrawal. If the visual stimuli had been removed first, there would have been a decrease in performance for three of the four subjects in this condition and it would have been necessary to reinstate the visual stimuli before examining the control of the other components. Thus, additional experimental manipulations over and above those discussed could have been necessary, depending on the order of component withdrawal.

In practice, both the stimulus control procedure and the sequential withdrawal provide a means of isolating factors that may maintain trained behaviors. An additional design option that also accomplishes this purpose is the partial withdrawal design.

Partial Withdrawal Design   Unlike the sequential withdrawal procedure, which can be used with reversal or multiple-baseline designs, partial withdrawal uniquely complements multiple-baseline designs. In essence, one or more treatment components is removed from one person, behavior, or situation after acquisition of target behaviors has been demonstrated using a multiple-baseline format. The partial withdrawal of a component, or of the entire treatment, from a single baseline provides an indication of what might happen across the remaining baselines if treatment was also removed. If the behavior is maintained after the withdrawal, evidence is available to suggest that similar results could be expected across the other baselines. Alternately, if a significant deterioration in responding is evident after the partial withdrawal, procedures can be implemented to facilitate maintenance in the first baseline and information is available regarding the remedial potential of the procedures across the remaining baselines.

Because examples of partial withdrawal procedures are not available in the communicative disorders literature, we will continue our discussion of the Carr et al. (1978) study of expressive sign acquisition to demonstrate this procedure. Recall that a multiple-baseline design across behaviors was employed in this study. A partial withdrawal could have been implemented by removing either a portion of treatment or the entire package for one baseline behavior. For example, a single stimulus item, such as "apple," could have been selected and one treatment component, the visual input, could have been withdrawn during maintenance probing. Based on previously presented results, it would appear that removal of the food item during probing would result in a decrease in rate of sign production for "apple" and this finding would suggest that removal of the other visual stimuli would have a similar effect on performance for the remaining food items. Therefore, the investigators would likely reintroduce the apple when probing for sign labeling of this item and they would continue to present the other items in order to facilitate generalization across time. As previously noted, a partial withdrawal may also be implemented by totally withdrawing treatment from one behavior, subject, or setting in a multiple-baseline study. A recent study by Schreibman and Carr (1978) can be used to demonstrate this procedure. The purpose of this study was to teach two echolalic children to produce an appropriate verbal response to previously echoed questions. A multiple-baseline design across two subjects, one retarded and one autistic, was used in this study. The target verbal response, "I don't know," was trained using a verbal prompt-fading procedure. That is, the experimenter initially modeled the target sentence after presenting a stimulus question (e.g., "Who are my friends?—I don't know"), reinforced echoed verbal responses, and then faded the prompt. Correct verbalizations were consequated throughout the treatment phase of the study. Results revealed that both children learned to produce the target utterance in response to questions that they had previously echoed. In addition, generalization was obtained to untrained questions and across examiners, and the effects of training were maintained on 1–month follow-up probes. Of particular interest for our purposes are the maintenance-probe procedures. Maintenance probes were administered using an intermixed-probe procedure. That is, trained and untrained questions were interspersed and appropriate responses to trained items were consequated. Verbal prompts were provided following incorrect responses to training questions but neither consequation nor prompts were provided following responses to untrained items. A partial withdrawal design for one of the two subjects in this study could have been implemented in the following manner.

For this subject, maintenance of trained responses would have been probed by having the experimenter present the stimulus question (e.g., Who are my friends?) and then waiting for the subject to respond. Consequation, repeats, and prompts would have been withdrawn and the experimenter would simply record the subject's responses. If the subject continued to respond at a high accuracy rate after removal of the treatment components, information would be available to suggest that similar results could be expected for the second subject. Given these findings, the experimenters might decide to withdraw the treatment package from the second subject because the first subject maintained a high level of responding without prompts and immediate consequation.

On the other hand, if removal of treatment variables resulted in a decrease in production of the target response, similar results would be expected for the second subject and prompts and consequation would not be withdrawn. In this case, the treatment variables might have been reinstated for subject 1 or remedial procedures could have been implemented to facilitate maintenance.

Although partial withdrawal provides a practical means of evaluating factors that contribute to response maintenance, data obtained by withdrawing treatment from one baseline may not be representative of what will happen across the remaining baselines if a similar withdrawal is implemented (Rusch and Kazdin, 1981). That is, factors that maintain target responding may differ across behaviors, subjects, and settings, and an investigator may not be able to predict accurately performance patterns of unmanipulated baselines from a single withdrawal. Similarly, if behavior is maintained after a partial withdrawal, an investigator cannot be certain which factor or factors are responsible for maintenance. It may be that components that are not withdrawn are maintaining the desired level of responding or, perhaps, contingencies in the natural environment are responsible for or contributing to maintenance.

In any event, if a partial withdrawal is not detrimental to one subject but results in a deterioration in performance for others, additional withdrawals will be needed to determine which components are exerting control over an individual subject's rate of responding. Rusch and Kazdin (1981) have suggested combining partial and sequential withdrawal procedures in order to "...predict, with increasing probability, the extent to which they are controlling the treatment environment as the progression of withdrawals is extended to other behaviors, subjects, or settings" (p. 136). Thus, if a partial withdrawal of treatment components results in deteriorating performance, sequential removal of treatment components could be attempted across other baselines to further assess stimulus control.

SUMMARY

Intervention researchers' interest in careful evaluation of treatments and the events composing them has encouraged development of designs that, although utilizing the basic components of within-subject designs, nevertheless arrange the components in various ways. Most of these designs are directed toward examination of treatments in a more comprehensive manner than allowed by the basic A-B-A-B and multiple-baseline designs.

The alternating-treatments design offers the researcher an opportunity to compare the effectiveness of two or more treatments. The interaction design allows careful evaluation of each component of a treatment package in relation to its contribution to the total package. In the changing-criterion design the researcher is able to follow changes in behavior as the subject gradually achieves a higher criterion level during treatment. Somewhat similarly, the multiple-probe design provides a framework for evaluating the contribution of steps or phases within a treatment program. Equally important are the various procedures designed to evaluate generalization, which were described in the final section of this chapter. These, beyond the basic designs, should facilitate identification of relevant and irrelevant factors in treatment and consequently contribute to improvement in intervention procedures.

Reflections

7

The ultimate purpose of applied communicative disorders research is to develop intervention techniques that can be readily incorporated into clinical practice. Within-subject experimental strategies are practical and clinically relevant and, as such, are suited to achieving this goal. The primary purpose of within-subject designs is to evaluate treatment effectiveness and promote clinically significant

changes in an individual's behavior. From a practical standpoint, the cost of coordinating and initiating a within-subject investigation is small, equipment needs are minimal, and few subjects are needed. Furthermore, some within-subject designs, such as the multiple-baseline design, can be incorporated into treatment programs without disrupting routine clinical activities. Thus, intrasubject designs provide an unobtrusive way to document the effectiveness of ongoing treatment and satisfy accountability needs. This benefit will become particularly important as third-party payment becomes increasingly dependent on documentation of quality clinical service. In the remainder of this chapter we consider several additional strengths of within-subject experimental strategies.

THE FLEXIBILITY OF WITHIN-SUBJECT DESIGNS

In the final analysis, proper use and interpretation of within-subject designs depends on an understanding of the basic logic of the applied behavioral approach to research (Kazdin, 1978; Johnston & Pennybacker, 1980). Principles of experimental control inherent in all within-subject studies, including continuous data collection, baseline-treatment comparisons, and intrasubject replications are far more critical than knowledge of any particular design. Hopefully, the designs that have been presented will not be applied in a "cookbook" fashion and previous discussion will serve as a framework for developing creative new intrasubject control procedures. There are, after all, no unalterable recipes for the conduct of experiments. Innumerable permutations and combinations of within-subject strategies are possible and "new" designs will be needed to solve problems that arise as we begin to interface within-subject methodology and communicative disorders research issues.

Design flexibility has been a hallmark of single-case experimental designs. Novel research strategies, such as the changing-criterion, alternating-treatments, and multiple-probe designs (Hartmann and Hall, 1976; Barlow and Hayes, 1979; Horner and Baer, 1978) have developed through creative application of applied behavioral logic. In addition, investigators have also combined designs in an attempt to enhance experimental control when a single strategy has proven insufficient. For example, Elbert and McReynolds (1978) used an A-B-A-B reversal design in combination with a multiple-baseline design in their study of articulation training and generalization. The primary purpose of this study was to explore the effects of context on generalization of trained phonemes. All five subjects consistently substituted / θ / for / s / during the baseline phase and they were trained to produce / s / correctly in syllable contexts during the first training condition. After all subjects reached a pre-established generalization criterion, a reversal procedure was implemented to demonstrate experimental control over the subjects' responses. Four of the five subjects reverted to their former error pattern in the generalization items during the reversal phase and, subsequently, / s / retraining was successful in reestablishing generative / s / responding. The multiple—baseline component of the study proved beneficial for demonstrating control for the subject who did not meet the generalization criterion in reversal training. This subject received training on a second phoneme, / r / , which had been held in baseline throughout previous phases of the study. Although the control sound had been consistently misarticulated before intervention, training was effective in establishing correct / r / production and experimental control was thereby demonstrated.

Another aspect of design flexibility has been previously mentioned but bears reiterating. Within-subject designs are uniquely versatile because repeated-measures data collection procedures provide information about changes in behavior *throughout* the entire length of an investigation. Whereas group researchers must often rely on pre- and post-treatment or, at best, occasional data collection, the applied behavioral researcher is kept in constant touch with the data. As a result, patterns of behavior change can be observed over time and abberrations in the data, such as intrasubject variability or change in slope or level, can be observed as they occur. More importantly, once a disturbing trend in data is identified, within-subject designs are flexible enough to be modified so that sources of variability can be brought under experimental control (Sidman, 1960; Hersen and Barlow, 1976). An example of the advantages of this type of design flexibility was previously noted in our discussion of a study by Roll (1973). The purpose of this study was to evaluate the effect of differential visual feedback on the degree of hypernasality exhibited by cleft palate children. Initially an A-B-A-B withdrawal design was planned in which visual feedback was presented contingent on the production of hypernasal sounds during the treatment phase and visual feedback was removed during a withdrawal phase. Although training was successful in decreasing the amount of hypernasality produced by the subjects, withdrawal of visual feedback did not result in the expected increase in hypernasality. Consequently, a feedback-reversal condition was initiated. In this condition the specific visual feedback provided for production of nasal and non-nasal sounds, red and white lights, respectively, was reversed. After the feedback-reversal phase, the amount of hypernasality produced approximated previous baseline levels. Thus, design flexibility permitted on-line adjustment and demonstration of experimental control.

In addition to the practical advantages presented above, design flexibility may contribute to the generalizability of within-subject findings. Hersen and Barlow (1976) note that design modifications that identify and control sources of variability extend generality by helping to define conditions under which treatment effects will be replicated. The generality of within-subject results will be further considered in the following discussion.

GENERALITY OF WITHIN-SUBJECT FINDINGS

Despite misconceptions, generality of within-subject findings to other clients, therapists, or conditions is not an inherent problem for within-subject research (Birnbrauer, 1981; Kazdin, 1981; Hersen and Barlow, 1976). As noted in Chapter 4, a proper series of direct and systematic replications can establish the generality of intrasubject research findings. Questions concerning the generality of intrasubject findings have, however, significantly retarded widespread acceptance of applied behavioral strategies (Hersen and Barlow, 1976) and a brief discussion of factors affecting the generality of findings is in order. Procedures for establishing generality have previously been considered and will not be reconsidered in the present discussion.

Generality in the group paradigm is based, to a large extent, on the process of random sampling of subjects. If a sample of subjects is randomly selected from an entire population, and the sample accurately represents the characteristics of the population, then results of studies on the sample are presumably generalizable to the entire population from which the sample was selected. In reality, practical problems involved in obtaining a random heterogeneous sample are nearly insurmountable. Researchers simply do not have access to a sufficient number of subjects to meet the randomization criteria, and representative samples, those that include all relevant characteristics of a population, are rarely available. Investigators usually opt for the practical solution of studying accessible subjects as they become available. As a result of nonrandom subject selection, statistical inferences from sample subjects to a population are not possible and inferences about individuals not

directly studied must be made on the basis of logical, nonstatistical considerations (Edgington, 1967; Edgar and Billingsley, 1974; Hersen and Barlow,
1976; Kazdin, 1981). Group investigators attempt to enhance the generality
of their findings by studying homogeneous, well-described subject groups.
Logical generality is improved when homogeneous subject groups are studied
because research consumers can determine if the group characteristics are
similar to those of an individual client. Logically, if a client closely resembles
a well described group of subjects for whom a given treatment was successful,
then one would have reason to infer that the treatment might also be efficacious for an individual client having similar characteristics. Alternately, as
samples become more heterogeneous, results are less generalizable to individual clients (Hersen and Barlow, 1976). In general, it is difficult to asess the
generality of group findings to individual clients because between-group
designs rely on statistical analysis of composite scores, usually a group
average, to make inferences about treatment effectiveness. Composite scores
obscure individual performance and intersubject variability (Sidman, 1960).

The controversy surrounding the generalizability of within-subject findings has continued, in part, because the results of studies of single individuals
are not generalizable. This is not, however, synonymous with saying that the
results of within-subject research have little or no generality. As we have
noted, replication is a powerful and accepted procedure for establishing the
generality of within-subject results. Furthermore, it is noteworthy that
replication is a powerful and accepted procedure for establishing the generality of within-subject results. Furthermore, it is noteworthy that within-
subject findings are routinely replicated within and across subjects. That is,
because of the small number of subjects studied and the need to establish the
reliability of findings, direct replication has become an integral component
of applied behavioral research. Controlled studies of single individuals are
becoming rare, and direct replication has become an implicit criterion for
publication in many applied journals. As with group research, generality of
within-subject findings is based on logical considerations. Direct replication
is available within intrasubject studies, however, and each replication
facilitates client generality.

Another aspect of within-subject research that facilitates generality is the
behavior-analytic insistence on clinical criteria for evaluating change (Baer,
1977b). Within-subject researchers generally insist on large, clinically significant change in behavior and less stringent statistical criteria are de-empha-
sized. Powerful treatment effects revealed in behavior-analytic studies are
likely to be highly replicable, perhaps more so than subtle effects revealed
through statistical analysis of group data. In the long run, powerful treatment effects will have a greater degree of generality than weaker effects.
Finally, Edgar and Billingsley (1974) provide another reason why generality

from within-subject findings may equal or surpass that of group studies. They note that the "more accurate delineation and precise control of subject characteristics" (p. 153) that typifies intensive designs may lead to statements of generality. We have already noted that heterogeneous subject populations and intersubject variability may make it difficult to determine the applicability of group findings to individual clients. Alternately, the operational specificity that characterizes within-subject research actually facilitates comparisons with other individuals and enhances logical generality to other clients.

To summarize, both within-subject and between-group findings can be used to establish generality and both approaches rely on logical, nonstatistical considerations to do so. Although it may be difficult to determine the generality of group-study results to individuals who are not directly studied, within-subject designs routinely include direct replication, a primary means of establishing client generality. In addition, clinical criteria and operational specificity, two fundamental aspects of within-subject research, also appear to facilitate client generality. Another important aspect of within-subject research, the breadth of problems explored with these designs, is discussed in the following section.

THE BREADTH OF WITHIN-SUBJECT DESIGNS

Applied behavioral researchers have frequently studied functional relationships between a single, well specified stimulus and a carefully defined subject response. This choice has, in part, reflected the belief that isolation of specific, powerful treatment variables is prerequisite to examining combined variables or treatment packages. Specific stimulus-response relationships are also frequently investigated in applied research for methodological reasons. The "one variable rule" of within-subject research precludes simultaneous manipulation of multiple variables across experimental phases. Whenever more than one variable is altered across phases, an investigator does not know which variable or combination of variables was responsible for changing subject behavior. Given the stringent control requirements and operational specificity evident in intrasubject research, it is perhaps not surprising that the breadth of this approach has not been recognized in the communicative disorders literature. It should be emphasized, however, that within-subject designs are not restricted to the examination of consequent events and simple stimulus-response relationships. Within-subject experimental strategies can be used to investigate a wide range of applied research issues and several of these are summarized in the following discussion.

One area of within-subject investigation not concerned with the effects of reinforcement is drug research. Withdrawal designs have been used to examine the effects of drugs on targeted behaviors and similar studies of communicative abilities can be envisioned. One might, for instance, use a withdrawal design to examine the effects of drug therapy on speech production of dysarthric individuals. Complex functional relationships between environment manipulation and communication have been examined with within-subject strategies. The complexity evident in Hart and Risley's (1974, 1975) research on "incidental teaching" of language to preschoolers can be cited in this respect. In each of these investigations small groups of subjects were studied simultaneously in a variety of preschool contexts and at various times during the day. In addition to revealing the complexity inherent in many within-subject investigations, this research demonstrates that applied behavioral designs have been used to study functional behaviors, in this case expansion of language skills, within natural environments. Moreover, topography of the responses trained, irrespective of the consequent events used in training, has served as the independent variable in articulation studies (Elbert and McReynolds, 1978; Rigor, 1980; Solomon, 1981). Within-subject research is increasingly expanding, moving from laboratory and analogue studies into a larger number of applied settings (Hayes et al., 1980).

Finally, the breadth of within-subject experimental strategies is evident in the wide range of topics that can be explored with these designs. Intrasubject designs are not, of course, appropriate for all research endeavors. They cannot, for example, be used to answer descriptive or actuarial questions and investigators interested in these issues must select a between-group design. Within-subject experimental strategies do, however, provide a powerful means of assessing functional relationships between treatment variables and communicative behaviors. In addition, these designs can be used to evaluate the contribution of separate components in a treatment package (interaction design), compare different treatments within the same individual (alternating-treatments design), examine individual steps within a treatment program (multiple-probe design) and explore the efficacy of shaping procedures (changing criterion design). Complex procedures, such as sequential or partial withdrawal, are available for examining the maintenance of trained behaviors. In short, all phases of the intervention process, acquisition, generalization, and maintenance, can be evaluated using within-subject experimental strategies. In time, communicative disorders researchers may use these designs to isolate treatment variables that, when used in combinations, will provide potent treatment packages. As this "technique building" process continues, we will add to the scientific basis for communicative disorders intervention.

References

Agras, W. S., Leitenberg, H., Barlow, D. H., and Thomson, L. E. 1969. Instructions and reinforcement in the modification of neurotic behavior. Am. J. Psychiatry 125:1435–1439.

American Speech-Language-Hearing Association 1980. Code of Ethics of the American Speech-Language-Hearing Association. Asha 22(1):41–43.

Azrin, N. H., and Holz, W. C. 1966. Punishment. In: W. K. Honig (ed.), Operant Behavior: Areas of Research and Application. Appleton-Century-Croft, New York. pp. 380–447.

Baer, D. M. 1977a. Reviewer's comment: just because it's reliable doesn't mean that you can use it. J. Appl. Behav. Anal. 10(1):117–119.

Baer, D. M. 1977b. Perhaps it would be better not to know everything. J. Appl. Behav. Anal. 10(1):167–172.

Baer, D. M., and Guess,D. 1971. Receptive training of adjectival inflections in mental retardates. J. Appl. Behav. Anal. 4: 129–139.

Baer, D. M., Wolf, M. M., and Risley, T. R. 1968. Some current dimensions of applied behavior analysis. J. Appl. Behav. Anal. 1(1):91–97.

Bakan, D. 1966. The test of significance in psychological research. Psychol. Bull. 66(6):423–437.

Baltaxe, C., and Simmons, J. Q. 1977. Bedtime soliloquies and linguistic competence in autism. J. Speech Hear. Disord. 42(3):376–393.

Barlow, D. H., and Hayes, S. C. 1979. Alternating treatments design: one strategy for comparing the effects of two treatments in a single subject. J. Appl. Behav. Anal. 12(2):199–210.

Benjamin, L. S. 1965. A special Latin square for the use of each subject as his own control. Psychometrika 30:499–513.

Bennett, C. W. 1974. Articulation training of two hearing-impaired girls. J. Appl. Behav. Anal. 7(3):439–445.

Bijou, S. W., Peterson, R. F., and Ault, M. H. 1968. A method to integrate descriptive and experimental field studies at the level of data and empirical concepts. J. Appl. Behav. Anal. 1(2):175–191.

Birkimer, J. D., and Brown, J. H. 1979a. A graphical judgment aid which summarizes obtained and chance reliability data and helps assess the believability of experimental effects. J. Appl. Behav. Anal. 12:523–534.

Birkimer, J. C., and Brown, J. H. 1979b. Back to basics: percentage agreement measures are adequate, but there are easier ways. J. Appl. Behav. Anal. 12:535–544.

Birnbrauer, J. S. 1981. External validity and experimental investigation of individual behavior. Anal. Interven. Devel. Disabil. 1:117–132.

Brady, D. O., and Smouse, A. D. 1978. A simultaneous comparison of three methods for language training with an autistic child: An experimental single case analysis. J. Autism Childhood Schizophren. 8(3):271–279.

Braukmann, C. J., Kirigin, K. A., and Wolf, M. M. 1976. Achievement Place: The researcher's perspective. Paper presented at the American Psychological Association, September, Washington, D. C.

Brodnitz, F. S. 1971. Vocal Rehabilitation. Whiting Press, Inc., Rochester, Minn.

Brookner, S. P., and Murphy, N. O. 1975. The use of a total communication approach with a nondeaf child: A case study. Lang. Speech Hear. Serv. Schools VI(3)131–153.

Browning, R. M. 1967. A same-subject design for simultaneous comparison of three reinforcement contingencies. Behav. Res. Therapy 5:237–243.

Browning, R. M., and Stover, D. O. 1971. Behavior modification in child treatment—an experimental and clinical approach. In: R. M. Browning and D. O. Stover (eds.), Behavior Modification in Child Treatment. Aldine Pub. Co., Chicago.

Campbell, D. T., and Stanley, J. C. 1966. Experimental and Quasi-experimental Designs for Research. Rand McNally & Company, Chicago.

Carr, E. G., Binkoff, J. A., Kologinsky, E., and Eddy, M. 1978. Acquisition of sign language by autistic children I: expressive labelling. J. Appl. Behav. Anal. 11:489–501.

Carver, R. P. 1978. The case against statistical significance testing. Harvard Ed. Rev. 48(3):378–399.

Clark, H. B., and Sherman, J. A. 1975. Teaching generative use of sentence answers to three forms of questions. J. Appl. Behav. Anal. 8:321–330.

Cone, T. D. 1979. Why the "I've got a better agreement measure" literature continues to grow: A commentary on two articles by Birkimer and Brown. J. Appl. Behav. Anal. 12:571–572.

Costello, J., and Ferrer, J. 1976. Punishment contingencies for the reduction of incorrect responses during articulation instruction. J. Commun. Disord. 9:43–61.

Costello, J., and Hairston, J. B. 1976. Concurrent modification of incorrect responses and off-task behavior occurring during articulation instruction. J. Commun. Disord. 9:175–190.

Costello, J. M., and Hurst, M. R. 1981. An analysis of the relationship among stuttering behaviors. J. Speech Hear. Res. 24(2):247–256.

Cuvo, A. J. 1979. Multiple-baseline design in instructional research: pitfalls of measurement and procedural advantages. J. Mental Defic. 84(3):219–228.

Daniel, B., and Guitar, B. 1978. EMG feedback and recovery of facial and speech gestures following neural anastomosis. J. Speech Hear. Disord. 43:9–20.

Davis, G. A. 1978. The Clinical Application of Withdrawal, Single-case Research Designs. Clinical Aphasiology Conference Proceedings. BRK Publishers, Minneapolis.

DeProspero, A., and Cohen, S. 1979. Inconsistent visual analyses of intrasubject data. J. Appl. Behav. Anal. 12(4):573–579.

Edgar, E., and Billingsley, F. 1974. Believability when N = 1. Psychol. Rec. 24:147–160.

Edgington, E. S. 1967. Statistical inference from N = 1 experiments. J. Psychol. 65:195–199.

Edgington, E. S. 1972. N = 1 experiments: Hypothesis testing. Canad. Psychol. 13:121–135.

Elbert, M., and McReynolds, L. V. 1975. Transfer of /r/ across contexts. J. Speech Hear. Disord. 40(3):380–387.

Elbert, M., and McReynolds, L. V. 1978. An experimental analysis of misarticulating children's generalization. J. Speech Hear. Res. 21:136–150.

Engel, D. C., and Groth, T. R. 1976. Case studies of the effect on carry-over of reinforcing postarticulation responses based on feedback. Lang. Speech Hear. Serv. Schools 7(2):93–101.

Fletcher, S. G. 1972. Contingencies for bioelectronic modification of nasality. J. Speech Hear. Disord. 47(3):329–345.

Frisch, S. A., and Schumaker, J. B. 1974. Training generalized receptive prepositions in retarded children. J. Appl. Behav. Anal. 7:611–621.

Furlong, M. J., and Wampold, B. E. 1981. Visual analysis of single-subject studies by school psychologists. Psychol. Schools 18:80–86.

Garcia, E. 1974. The training and generalization of a conversational speech form in nonverbal retardates. J. Appl. Behav. Anal. 7:137–149.

Garcia, E. E., and DeHaven, E. D. 1974. Use of operant techniques in the establishment and generalization of language: A review and analysis. Am. J. Mental Defic. 79(2):169–178.

Gentile, J. R., Roden, A. H., and Klein, R. D. 1972. An analysis of variance model for the intrasubject replication design. J. Appl. Behav. Anal. 5:193–198.

Gresham, F. M. 1979. Comparison of response cost and timeout in a special setting. J. Spec. Ed. 13(2):199–208.

Guess, D., and Baer, D. M. 1973. Some experimental analyses of linguistic development in institutionalized retarded children. In: Lahey (ed.), The Modification of Language Behavior. Charles C. Thomas, Springfield, Ill.

Guess, D., Keogh, W., and Sailor, W. 1978. Generalization of speech and language behavior measurement and training tactics. In: Schiefelbusch (ed.), Bases of Language Intervention. University Park Press, Baltimore.

Guilford, J. P. 1954. Psychometric Methods. (2nd ed.) McGraw-Hill Book Co., New York.

Guitar, B. 1975. Reduction of stuttering frequency using analog electromyographic feedback. J. Speech Hear. Res. 18:672–685.

Haase, R. F., and Tepper, D. T. 1972. Non-verbal components of empathetic communication. J. Counsel. Psychol. 19:417–424.

Hall, R. V., and Fox, R. G. 1977. Changing criterion designs: an alternate applied behavior analysis procedure. In: C. C. Etzel, G. M. LeBlanc, and D. M. Baer (eds.), New Developments in Behavioral Research: Theory, Method and Application. Lawrence Erlbaum Assoc., Hillsdale, N.J.

Handelman, J. S. 1981. Transfer of verbal responses across instructional settings by autistic-type children. J. Speech Hear. Disord. 46:69–76.

Hanna, R., Wilfing, F., and McNeill, B. 1975. A biofeedback treatment for stuttering. J. Speech Hear. Disord. 40:270–273.

Harris, F. C., and Ciminero, A. R. 1978. The effect of witnessing consequences on the behavioral recordings of experimental observers. J. Appl. Behav. Anal. 11(4):513–521.

Harris, F. C., and Lahey, B. B. 1978. A method for combining occurrence and nonoccurence interobserver agreement scores. J. Appl. Behav. Anal. 11(4):523–527.

Harris, S. L. 1975. Teaching language to nonverbal children—with emphasis on problems of generalization. Psychol. Bull. 82(4):565–580.

Hart, B., and Risley, T. R. 1974. Using preschool materials to modify the language of disadvantaged children. J. Appl. Behav. Anal. 7(2):243–256.

Hart, B., and Risley, T. R. 1975. Incidental teaching of language in the pre-school. J. Appl. Behav. Anal. 8:411–420.

238   Single-Subject Experimental Designs

Hart, B., and Risley, T. R. 1980. In vivo language intervention: unanticipated general effects. J. Appl. Behav. Anal. 13:407–432.

Hartmann, D. P. 1974. Forcing square pegs into round holes: some comments on "Analysis of Variance Model for the Intrasubject Replication Design." J. Appl. Behav. Anal. 7(4):635–638.

Hartmann, D. P. 1977. Considerations in the choice of interobserver reliability estimates. J. Appl. Behav. Anal. 10(1):103–116.

Hartmann, D. P., and Hall, R. V. 1976. The changing criterion design. J. Appl. Behav. Anal. 9(4):527–532.

Hartmann, D. P., Gottman, T. M., Jones, R. R., Gardner, W., Kazdin, A. E., and Vaught, R. 1980. Interrupted time-series analysis and its application to behavioral data. J. Appl. Behav. Anal. 13:543–559.

Hawkins, R. P., and Dotson, V. A. 1975. Reliability scores that delude: An Alice in Wonderland trip through the misleading characteristics of interobserver agreement scores in interval recording. In: E. Ramp, and G. Semb, (eds.), Behavior Analysis: Areas of Research and Application. Prentice Hall, Inc., New Jersey.

Hawkins, R. P., and Farby, B. D. 1979. Applied behavior analysis and interobserver reliability: A commentary on two articles by Birkimer and Brown. J. Appl. Behav. Anal. 12(4):545–552.

Hayes, S. C., Rincover, A., and Solnick, J. V. 1980. The technical drift of applied behavior analysis. J. Appl. Behav. Anal. 13(2):275–285.

Hegde, M. N. 1980. An experimental clinical analysis of grammatical and behavioral distinctions between verbal auxiliary and copula. J. Speech Hear. Res. 23:864–877.

Hegde, M. N., and Gierut, J. 1979. The operant training and generalization of pronouns and a verb form in a language delayed child. J. Commun. Disord. 12:23–34.

Hegde, M. N., Noll, M. J., and Pecora, R. 1979. A study of some factors affecting generalization of language training. J. Speech Hear. Disord. 44:301–320.

Hersen, M., and Barlow, D. H. 1976. Single Case Experimental Designs—Strategies for Studying Behavior Change. Pergamon Press Inc., New York.

Heward, W. L., and Eachus, H. T. 1979. Acquisition of adjectives and adverbs in sentences written by hearing impaired and aphasic children. J. Appl. Behav. Anal. 12(3):391–400.

Holbrook, A. 1980. An instrumental approach to the assessment and remediation of speech disorders. In: L. P. Ince, (ed.), Behavioral Psychology In Rehabilitation Medicine: Clinical Applications. Williams and Wilkins, Baltimore.

Hopkins, B. L. 1979. Proposed conventions for evaluating observer reliability: A commentary on two articles by Birkimer and Brown. J. Appl. Behav. Anal. 12:561–564.

Hopkins, B. L., and Hermann, J. A. 1977. Evaluating interobserver reliability of interval data. J. Appl. Behav. Anal. 10(1):121–126.

Horner, R. D., and Baer, D. M. 1978. Multiple-probe technique: A variation of the multiple baseline. J. Appl. Behav. Anal. 11(1):189–196.

Ingham, R. J. 1975. A comparison of covert and overt assessment procedures in stuttering therapy outcome evaluation. J. Speech Hear. Res. 18(2):346–354.

Jackson, D. A., and Wallace, R. F. 1974. The modification and generalization of voice loudness in a fifteen-year-old retarded girl. J. Appl. Behav. Anal. 7:461–471.

Johnson, M. C., and Kaye, J. H. 1976. Acquisition of lipreading in a deaf multihandicapped child. J. Speech Hear. Disord. 41(2):226–232.

Johnson, S. M., and Bolstad, O. D. 1973. Methodological issues in naturalistic observation: Some problems and solutions for field research. In: L. A. Hamerlynch, L. C. Handy, and E. I. Mash (eds.), pp. 7–67. Behavior Change: Methodology, Concepts, and Practice. Research Press, Champaign, Ill.

Johnston, J. M., and Johnston, G. T. 1972. Modification of consonant speech-sound articulation in young children. J. Appl. Behav. Anal. 5:233–246.

Johnston, J. M., and Pennypacker, H. S. 1980. Strategies and Tactics of Human Behavioral Research. Lawrence Erlbaum, Assoc., Pub., Hillsdale, N. J.

Jones, R. J., and Azrin, N. H. 1969. Behavioral engineering: Stuttering as a function of stimulus duration during speech synchronization. J. Appl. Behav. Anal. 2:223–230.

Jones, R. R., Vaught, R. S., and Weinrott, M. 1977. Time-series analysis in operant research. J. Appl. Behav. Anal. 10(1):151–166.

Jones, R. R., Weinrott, M. R., and Vaught, R. S. 1978. Effects of serial dependency on agreement between visual and statistical inference. J. Appl. Behav. Anal. 11(2):277–283.

Kazdin, A. E., 1973. Methodological and assessment considerations in evaluating reinforcement programs in applied settings. J. Appl. Behav. Anal. 6(3):517–531.

Kazdin, A. E. 1975a. The impact of applied behavior analysis on diverse areas of research. J. Appl. Behav. Anal. 8(2):213–229.

Kazdin, A. E. 1975b. Characteristics and trends in applied behavior analysis. J. Appl. Behav. Anal. 8(3):332.

Kazdin, A. E. 1976. Statistical Analyses for Single-case Experimental Designs. In: Michel Hersen and David Barlow (eds.), Single Case Experimental Designs—Strategies for Studying Behavior Change. Pergamon Press, New York.

Kazdin, A. E. 1977a. Artifacts, bias, and complexity of assessment: The ABCs of reliability. J. Appl. Behav. Anal. 10(1):141–150.

Kazdin, A. E. 1977b. Methodology of applied behavior. In: T. A. Brigham and A. E. Catania (eds.), Social and Instructional Processes: Foundations and Application. John Wiley and Sons, New York.

Kazdin, A. 1977c. Assessing the clinical or applied importance of behavior change through social validation. Behav. Mod. 1(4):427–452.

Kazdin, A. E. 1978. Methodological and interpretive problems of single-case experimental designs. J. Consult. Clin. Psychol. 46(4):629–642.

Kazdin, A. E. 1979. Unobtrusive measures in behavioral assessment. J. Appl. Behav. Anal. 12:713–724.

Kazdin, A. E. 1980. Sources of artifact and bias. Research Design in Clinical Psychology, Harper and Row, New York.

Kazdin, A. E. 1981. External validity and single-case experimentation: Issues and limitations (A response to J. S. Birnbrauer). Anal. Interven. Devel. Disabil. 1:133–144.

Kazdin, A. E., and Geesey, S. 1977. Simultaneous-treatment design comparisons of the effects of earning reinforcers for one's peers versus for oneself. Behav. Ther. 8:682–693.

Kazdin, A. E., and Hartmann, D. P. 1978. The simultaneous-treatment design. Behav. Ther. 9:912–922.

Kazdin, A. E., and Kopel, S. A. 1975. On resolving ambiguities of the multiple baseline design: problems and recommendations. Behav. Ther. 6:601–608.

Kearns, K., and Salmon, S. An experimental analysis of auxiliary and copula verb generalization. J. Speech Hear. Disord. (In press).

Kelly, M. B. 1977. A review of the observational data-collection and reliability procedures reported in the Journal of Applied Behavior Analysis. J. Appl. Behav. Anal. 10(1):97–101.

Kent, R. N., and Foster, S. L. 1977. Direct observational procedures: Methodological issues in naturalistic settings. In: A. R. Ciminero, K. S. Calhoun, and H. E. Adams, (eds.), Handbook of Behavioral Assessment. John Wiley and Sons, New York.

Kent, R. N., Kanowitz, J., O'Leary, K. D., and Cheiken, M. 1977. Observer reliability as a function of circumstances of assessment. J. Appl. Behav. Anal. 10(2):317–324.

Kent, R. N., O'Leary, K. D., Diament, C., and Dietz, A. 1974. Expectation biases in observational evaluation of therapeutic change. J. Consult. Clin. Psychol. 42:774–780.

Koegel, R. L., Egel, A. L., and Williams, J. A. 1980. Behavioral contrast and generalization across settings in the treatment of autistic children. J. Exp. Psychol. 30:422–437.

Kotkin, R. A., Simpson, S. B., and DeSanto, D. 1978. The effect of sign language on picture naming in two retarded girls possessing normal hearing. J. Mental Defic. Res. 22:19–25.

Kratochwill, T. R. (ed.). 1978. Single Subject Research—Strategies for Evaluating Change. Academic Press, New York.

Kratochwill, T. R., and Brody, G. H. 1978. Single subject designs—A perspective on the controversy over employing statistical inference and implications for research and training in behavior modification. Behav. Mod. 2(3):291–307.

Kratochwill, T. R., and Levin, J. R. 1980. On the applicability of various data analysis procedures to the simultaneous and alternating treatment designs in behavior therapy research. Behav. Assess. 2:353–360.

Kratochwill, T. R., and Wetzel, R. J. 1977. Observer agreement, credibility, and judgment: Some considerations in presenting observer agreement data. J. Appl. Behav. Anal. 10(1):133–139.

Leitenberg, H. 1973. The use of single-case methodology in psychotherapy research. J. Abnormal Psychol. 82(1):87–101.

Lindquist, E. F. 1953. Design and Analysis of Experiments in Psychology and Education. Houghton Mifflin Co., Boston.

Ling, D. 1976. Speech and the Hearing Impaired Child: Theory and Practice. The Alexander Graham Bell Association for the Deaf, Inc., Washington, D.C.

Lutzker, J. R., and Sherman, J. A. 1974. Producing generative sentence usage by imitation and reinforcement procedures. J. Appl. Behav. Anal. 7(3):447–460.

McNeill, M. R., and Prescott, T. E. 1978. Revised Token Test. University Park Press, Baltimore.

McReynolds, L. V. 1980. Co-articulation and context. Paper presented at the American Speech-Language-Hearing Convention, Detroit, Mich.

Mann, R. A., and Baer, D. M. 1971. The effects of receptive language training on articulation. J. Appl. Behav. Anal. 4(4):291–298.

Marholin, D., II., Siegel, L. J., and Phillips, D. 1976. Treatment and transfer: A search for empirical procedures. In: M. Hersen, R. M. Eisler, and P. M. Miller (eds.). Progress In Behavior Modification. Vol. III. Academic Press, New York.

Martin, R. R., and Siegel, G. M. 1966. The effects of simultaneously punishing stuttering and rewarding fluency. J. Speech Hear. Res. 9(3):466–475.

Mash, E. J., and McElwee, J. T. D. 1974. Situational effects on observer accuracy: Behavior predictability, prior experience, and complexity of coding categories. Child Develop. 45:367–377.

Michael, J. 1974a. Statistical inference for individual organism research: Some reactions to a suggestion by Gentile, Roden, and Klein. J. Appl. Behav. Anal. 7(4):627–628.

Michael, J. 1974b. Statistical inference for individual organism research: Mixed blessing or curse? J. Appl. Behav. Anal. 7:647–653.

Murdock, T. Y., Garcia, E., and Hardman, M. L. 1977. Generalizing articulation training with trainable mentally retarded subjects. J. Appl. Behav. Anal. 10:717–733.

Murphy, R. J., and Bryan, A. J. 1980. Multiple-baseline and multiple-probe designs: Practical alternatives for special education assessment and evaluation. J. Special Ed. 14(3):325–335.

Murphy, R., Doughty, N., and Nunes, D. 1979. The multielement designs: An alternative to reversal and multiple baseline evaluation strategies. Ment. Retard. 17:23–27.

Neale, J. M., and Liebert, R. M. 1973. Science and Behavior. Prentice-Hall, Englewood Cliffs, N.J.

Netsell, R., and Cleeland, C. S. 1973. Modification of lip hypertonia in dysarthria using EMG feedback. J. Speech Hear. Disord. 38(1):131–140.

Nober, E. H. 1967. Articulation of the deaf. Exceptional Child 33:611–621.

O'Brien, F., Azrin, N. H., and Henson, K. 1969. Increased communications of chronic mental patients by reinforcement and by response priming. J. Appl. Behav. Anal. 2:23–29.

O'Leary, K. D., and Drabman, R. 1971. Token reinforcement programs in the classroom: A review. Psychol. Bull. 75:379–398.

O'Leary, K. D., Kent, R. N., and Kanowitz, J. 1975. Shaping data collection congruent with experimental hypotheses. J. Appl. Behav. Anal. 8:43–51.

Parsonson, B. S., and Baer, D. M. 1978. The analysis and presentation of graphic data. In: T. R. Kratochwill (ed.). Single Subject Research Strategies for Evaluating Change. Academic Press, New York.

Porch, B E. 1971. The Porch Index of Communicative Ability. Consulting Psychologists Press, Palo Alto, California.

Powell, J., Martindale, A., and Kulp, S. 1975. An evaluation of time-sample measures of behavior. J. Appl. Behav. Anal. 8(4):463–469.

Reid, D. H., and Hurlbut, B. 1977. Teaching non-vocal communication skills to multihandicapped retarded adults. J. Appl. Behav. Anal. 10(4):591–603.

Reid, J. B. 1970. Reliability Assessment of observation data: A possible methodological problem. Child Develop. 41:1143–1150.

Repp, A. C., Roberts, D. M., Slack, D. T., Repp, C. F., and Berkler, M. S. 1976. A comparison of frequency interval and time-sampling methods of data collection. J. Appl. Behav. Anal. 9:501–508.

Revusky, S. H. 1967. Some statistical treatments compatible with individual organism methodology. J. Exp. Anal. Behav. 10:319–330.

Rigor, S. M. 1980. An experimental analysis of articulation generalization as a function of elicitation method and sampling context during articulation training. Masters Thesis, University of Kansas.

Roll, D. L. 1973. Modification of nasal resonance in cleft-palate children by informative feedback. J. Appl. Behav. Anal. 6(3):397–403.

Romanczyk, R. G., Kent, R. N., Diament, C., and O'Leary, K. D. 1973. Measuring the reliability of observational data: A reactive process. J. Appl. Behav. Anal. 1:175–184.

Roodenberg, W. F., and Smeets, P. M. 1980. Establishing respondent nonspeech communication in a retarded quadriplegic woman. Behav. Engineer. 6(2):91–100.

Rosenbaum, M. S., and Breiling, J. 1976. The development and functional control of reading—comprehension behavior. J. Appl. Behav. Anal. 9(3):323–333.

Rosenthal, R. 1979. The "File Drawer Problem" and tolerance for null results. Psychol. Bull. 86(3):638–641.

Rusch, F. R., and Kazdin, A. E. 1981. Toward a methodology of withdrawal designs for the assessment of response maintenance. J. Appl. Behav. Anal. 14:131–140.

Sailor, W. 1971. Reinforcement and generalization of productive plural allomorphs in two retarded children. J. Appl. Behav. Anal. 4:305–310.

Salzinger, K. 1967. The problem of response class in verbal behavior. In: K. Salzinger and S. Salzinger (eds.). Research in Verbal Behavior and Some Neurophysical Implications. Academic Press, New York.

Sanson-Fisher, R. W., Poole, A. D., and Dunn, J. 1980. An empirical method for determining an appropriate interval length for recording behavior. J. Appl. Behav. Anal. 13:493–500.

Schreibman, L., and Carr, E. G. 1978. Elimination of echolalic responding to questions through the training of a generalized verbal response. J. Appl. Behav. Anal. 11(4):453–463.

Sidman, M. 1960. Tactics Of Scientific Research—Evaluating Experimental Data in Psychology. Basic Books, Inc., New York.

Siegel, S. 1956. Nonparametric Statistics For The Behavioral Sciences. McGraw-Hill Book Co., New York.

Silverman, F. H. 1977. Research Design In Speech Pathology And Audiology. Prentice Hall, Englewood Cliffs, N.J.

Smith, Jr., N. C. 1970. Replication studies: A neglected aspect of psychology research. Am. Psychol. 25:970–975.

Solomon, L. 1981. Articulation generalization in hearing impaired children. Unpublished dissertation. University of Kansas.

Spradlin, J. K., Karlan, G. R., and Wetherby, B. 1976. Behavior analysis, behavior modification, and developmental disabilities. In: L. Lloyd (ed.). Communication Strategies and Intervention Strategies. University Park Press, Baltimore. pp. 225–263.

Starkweather, W. C. 1971. The case against base rate comparisons in stuttering experimentation. J. Commun. Disord. 4:247–258.

Stokes, T. F., and Baer, D. M. 1977. An implicit technology of generalization. J. Appl. Behav. Anal. 10(2):349–367.

Sulzer-Azaroff, B. and Mayer, C. 1977. Applying Behavior Analysis Procedures With Children and Youth. Holt, Rinehart and Winston, New York. pp. 487–499.

Thompson, Jr., G. A., Iwata, B. A., and Poynter, H. 1979. Operant control of pathological tongue thrust in spastic cerebral palsy. J. Appl. Behav. Anal. 12(3):325–333.

Thoresen, C. E., and Elashoff, J. D. 1974. "An analysis-of-variance model for intra-subject replication design": Some additional comments. J. Appl. Behav. Anal. 4:639–641.

Thorndike, R. L., and Hagen, E. P. 1977. Measurement and Evaluation In Psychology. (4th ed.). John Wiley & Sons, New York.

Tucker, D. J., and Berry, G. W. 1980. Teaching severely multihandicapped students to put on their own hearing aids. J. Appl. Behav. Anal. 13(1):65–75.

Ulman, J. D., and Sulzer-Azaroff, B. 1975. Multielement baseline design in educational research. In: E. Ramp and G. Semb (eds.). Behavior Analysis: Areas of Research and Application. Prentice Hall, Englewood Cliffs, N. J.

Van Houten, R. 1979. Social validation: The evolution of standards of competency for target behaviors. J. Appl. Behav. Anal. 12(4):581–591.

Ventry, I. M., and Schiavetti, N. 1980. Evaluating Research In Speech Pathology and Audiology, Addison-Wesley, Reading, Mass.

Wahler, R. G. 1969. Setting generality: Some specific and general effects of child behavior therapy. J. Appl. Behav. Anal. 2:239–246.

Wahler, R. G., Berland, R. M., and Coe, T. D. 1979. Generalization processes in child behavior change. In: B. B. Lahey and A. E. Kazdin, (eds.). Advances In Clinical Psychology, Vol. 2. Plenum Press, New York.

Wampold, B. E., and Furlong, M. J. 1981. The heuristics of visual inference. Behav. Assess. 3:79–92.

Welch, S. J., and Pear, J. J. 1980. Generalization of naming responses to objects in the natural environment as a function of training stimulus modality with retarded children. J. Appl. Behav. Anal. 13:629–643.

Wertz, R. T. 1978. Neuropathologies of speech and language: An introduction to patient management. In: D. F. Johns (ed.) Clinical Management of Neurogenic Communicative Disorders. Little Brown & Co., Boston, Mass.

Wheeler, A. J., and Sulzer, B. 1970. Operant training and generalization of a verbal response form in a speech deficient child. J. Appl. Behav. Anal. 3:139–147.

White, O. R. 1972. The split-middle: A quickie method of trend analysis. Paper presented at Regions/Resource Center for Handicapped Children, Eugene, Oregon.

Wildman, II, R. W., and Wildman, R. W. 1975. The generalization of behavior modification procedures: A review—with special emphasis on classroom applications. Psychol. Schools 12(4):432-438.

Winer, B. J. 1962. Statistical Principles in Experimental Design. McGraw-Hill Book Co., New York.

Wolf, M. M. 1978. Social validity: The case for subjective measurement or how applied behavior analysis is finding its heart. J. Appl. Behav. Anal. 11(2):203–214.

Wolf, M., and Risley, T. R. 1971. Reinforcement: Applied research. In: R. Glaser (ed.). The Nature of Reinforcement. Academic Press, New York.

Yelton, A. R., Wildman, B. G., and Erickson, M. T. 1977. A probability-based formula for calculating interobserver agreement. J. Appl. Behav. Anal. 10(1):127–131.

Author Index

Subject Index